Casting and Mending

Casting
AND
Mending

How therapeutic

fly fishing heals shattered

minds and bodies

Patrick M. Scanlon

RIT Press
Rochester, N.Y.

Published and distributed by:

RIT Press
90 Lomb Memorial Drive
Rochester, New York 14623
http://ritpress.rit.edu

ISBN 978-1-939125-97-2 (print)
ISBN 978-1-939-125-98-9 (e-book)

Printed in the U.S.A.

Cover design: Eric C. Wilder

Library of Congress Cataloging-in-Publication Data

Names: Scanlon, Patrick McRae, 1952- author.
Title: Casting and mending : how therapeutic fly fishing heals shattered
   minds and bodies / Patrick M. Scanlon.
Description: Rochester, NY : RIT Press, [2022] | Includes bibliographical references. | Summary:
   "The notion that fishing is about more than catching fish, that it offers tranquility, reflection,
   and recovery, is at the heart of scores of programs across the United States that use fly fishing
   to promote physical and emotional healing. Healing for people with cancer, for veterans with
   Post-Traumatic Stress Disorder and physical disabilities, and for those in recovery from drug and
   alcohol addiction. Casting and Mending: How therapeutic fly fishing heals shattered minds and
   bodies tells the story of several of these programs, including the voices of breast cancer patients,
   veterans, and recovering addicts as they reflect on the often life-changing and life-affirming experience of fly fishing. Casting and Mending also traces fishing in history and popular culture as a
   source of solace and redemption; explores the science of the healing effects of nature; and makes
   a case for fly fishing as an instance of "flow," an optimal experience that leaves a person stronger,
   more confident, and refreshed"-- Provided by publisher.
Identifiers: LCCN 2022017016 (print) | LCCN 2022017017 (ebook) | ISBN
   9781939125972 (paperback) | ISBN 9781939125989 (ebook)
Subjects: LCSH: Fly fishing--Anecdotes. | Mind and body therapies.
Classification: LCC SH456 .S28 2022 (print) | LCC SH456 (ebook) | DDC
   799.12/4--dc23/eng/20220617
LC record available at https://lccn.loc.gov/2022017016
LC ebook record available at https://lccn.loc.gov/2022017017

To Joanne

And it shall come to pass, that every thing that liveth, which moveth, whithersoever the rivers shall come, shall live: and there shall be a very great multitude of fish, because these waters shall come thither: for they shall be healed; and every thing shall live whither the river cometh.
—Ezekiel 47:9 KJV

Table of Contents

Preface

Fly fishing has a reputation for being exceptional, transcendent, even mystical. One author, Harry Middleton, calls the sport a "way of sinking into the press of time, into the current of all moments that ever were, are, or will be." A lifelong fly fisherman myself, I've never been able to take this attitude altogether seriously, even if I haven't swung all the way to the perspective of Jack Handey, as expressed in one of his "Deep Thoughts": "Marta says the interesting thing about fly fishing is that it's two lives connected by a thin strand. Come on, Marta. Grow up." While I'm an avid fly fisherman, I know that it can be the subject of a good deal of baloney.

So I was skeptical when I began to learn about the many programs throughout the United States and elsewhere that use fly fishing as a form of therapy for damaged bodies and minds. I couldn't help but wonder: Do participants in these programs actually realize physical and emotional benefits, and is there scientific proof? Or are such programs simply another instance of the Zen of fly fishing?

To get some firsthand experience, I wangled an invitation to observe the fishing portion of a Casting for Recovery Retreat on the Salmon River in western New York, a couple hours' drive from where I live. I watched as fourteen women with breast cancer went fly fishing, assisted by dozens of volunteers. What I saw and heard from the women that day suggested a life-changing experience, one I was eager to learn more about. Since then, I've spent time embedded with other therapeutic fly-fishing programs and interviewed scores of professionals, volunteers, and, most importantly, participants. I also immersed myself in relevant literature concerning health and recreation, the therapeutic benefits of green spaces, and more. The result is this book.

Is fly fishing therapeutic? *Casting and Mending* answers that question with a resounding, "Yes." It begins by tracing the history of fly fishing as a meditative, restorative pursuit. Next, it explores the healing benefits of fly-fishing programs for women with breast cancer (Part 1), veterans and active military members suffering from Post-Traumatic Stress Disorder and physical injuries (Part 2), and those in recovery from alcohol and drug addiction (Part 3). Each section concludes with the voices of therapeutic fly-fishing program participants. Part 4, "How Fly Fishing Heals," reviews scientific research into how physical and mental health are improved by being in natural environments, particularly those where fly fishing takes place, and makes a case for the "flow" of fly fishing by drawing on the groundbreaking work on optimal experience by Mihaly Csikszentmihalyi.

The book may be of value to fly fishers as well as anyone interested in the physical and mental health benefits of fly fishing specifically and outdoor activities generally. *Casting and Mending* may be particularly illuminating for those involved in complementary medicine, as they will learn of another potential treatment for a host of mental and physical conditions. I hope they will see therapeutic fly fishing as an opportunity to expand their toolkits. Finally, all readers will come to see that fly fishing truly can be about more than just catching fish.

A word about the title, whose double meaning may not be evident to the non-angler: When fly fishers cast a line across and onto a stream, the irregular flow makes sinuous what was momentarily straight as a tightrope. A length of the line bows downstream in a rush, drawing the leader with it like cracking the whip, and drags the imitation in a way no insect moves. To entice a trout, anglers want the fly to drift naturally, so they snap the rod upward to lift the line off the surface and, with an upstream jog of the wrist, shape the line into an arc on the water above the fly, creating slack. This is called mending the line.

Mend: repair, restore, put right. Recover. Heal.

Chapter 1

Diverter of Sadness and Calmer of Unquiet Thoughts

How fly fishing became therapeutic

Angling was after tedious Study, a rest to his mind, a chearer [sic] of his spirits, a diverter of sadness, a calmer of unquiet thoughts, a moderator of passions, a procurer of contentedness; and that it begat habits of peace and patience in those that profess'd and practis'd it.
—Izaak Walton, *The Compleat Angler*

Whenever I was along the river, fishing its bright water, I let myself go, emptied my head, let the moving river soothe my ache for contact and connection, ease my heart's ancient longing for its legacy of wildness.
—Harry Middleton, *The Bright Country: A Fisherman's Return to Trout, Wild Water, and Himself*

Dozens of programs throughout the United States and elsewhere use fly fishing for physical and emotional healing. These include, for cancer survivors: Casting for Recovery, Casting for Hope, Hope on the Rise, and Reel Recovery; for disabled veterans and active military personnel: Project Healing Waters Fly Fishing, Rivers of Recovery, and OASIS (Outdoor Adventures for Sacrifice in Service); and for recovering addicts, Four Circles Recovery Center and Rainbow's End Recovery Center. Fly fishing is even the centerpiece of several private psychological counseling practices. "Therapeutic fly fishing" appears so often in the literature on complementary medicine that it has earned an initialism, TFF.

Casting for Recovery summarizes the benefits of TFF this way:

> On a physical level, the gentle, rhythmic motion of fly casting is similar to exercises often prescribed after surgery or radiation to promote soft tissue stretching. On an emotional level, women are given the opportunity to experience a new activity in a safe environment amongst a supportive group of peers. The retreats provide resources to help address quality of life issues after a breast cancer diagnosis, and a new outlet–fly fishing–as a reprieve from the everyday stresses and challenges of their cancer.

Project Healing Waters similarly promotes fly fishing's therapeutic effects on body and soul:

> The motions involved in fly tying, casting, and fishing provide physical therapy for torn and tattered bodies. Damaged hands respond nicely to fly tying; injured arms, shoulders, and backs get a wholesome and much-needed workout during casting, mending, and retrieving. Even more important, minds and hearts are refreshed by the tranquility of moving waters.

Claims made for the healing powers of fly fishing reflect popular images of the sport reaching back at least to the seventeenth century. Fly fishing takes place outdoors in tranquil settings along gently flowing, calm-inducing streams. It requires practice that is gratifying and concentration that is distracting. Think of the novice who masters that metronomic sweep of the fly rod, the sense of accomplishment at watching the line loop out over the water, perhaps delivering a fly she tied herself, and landing a trout.

The many therapeutic fly-fishing programs that have sprung up around the country over the past two decades are part of a centuries-long tradition that sees the sport as a nearly mystical connection between nature and ourselves. The high point in popular culture may have come in 1992 when Robert Redford brought *A River Runs Through It* to the big screen, but fly fishing has a long history as a source of tranquility, reflection, solace, and recovery.

In the opening sentence of his book *The Science of Fly-fishing*, Stan Ulanski writes, "The sport of fly-fishing has often been embellished in hyperbole." Perhaps he was thinking of authors who depict fly fishing as transcendent, spiritual—numinous. They compose extravagant testimonials to the sport's interconnections with the natural world, deep time, and the collective unconscious. In the hands of the best of these writers, the prose can be enchanting, as in this passage by the late Harry Middleton:

> Angling, for me, is about a lot more than fishing. It is one way of sinking into the press of time, into the current of all moments that ever were, are, or will be, thinking, as the river's current tugs at my calves and thighs, about such lucky coincidences as wild water and trout and me, the awkward mammal with his big brain and evolving, menacing consciousness, casting for rising trout, for those dim memories and worn connections to everything that was and is, the world of imperfections and luck and successful accidents, fortunate divergence.

This is to say, there is fishing, and there is fly fishing. While the spin-caster stands on shore or sits in a boat, the fly fisher plants himself in the stream, attuned to the motion of water, the life cycle of aquatic insects, and the habits of trout. The former throws a lure that pulls line off a spool. The latter creates graceful loops in a fly line to present a weightless imitation to a rising fish. One is relaxing; the other is engaging with the natural world on its own terms.

Overstated or not, fly fishing has earned a special place in the popular imagination. It is particularly strongly linked to spirituality and self-discovery, to a Zen-like state of meditation-in-nature. The spirituality of fly fishing certainly is real for the authors of *Fly-fishing—the sacred art: Casting a fly as a spiritual practice*, one of whom writes, "I experience living, breathing, radical life-giving God in each and every wisp of wind, riffle, deer sighting, and shimmer of flashing trout." Sentiments like that are common in writing about fly fishing, which has a reputation for offering anglers a connection to something larger than themselves and a path to personal well-being. These notions are fundamental to much therapeutic fly fishing. But how did that happen? How did we get from fishing to "sinking into the press of time" and finding peace and enlightenment through the act of casting a fly line?

Human beings have been catching fish for at least 40,000 years. Fish hooks made of bone have been found that are about 20,000 years old. In 1913, a Finnish farmer discovered a fishing net, made of willow fibers and approximately 100 feet by 5 feet, which has been carbon dated to 8300 B.C.

People also have taken fish with weirs and harpoons and their bare hands. An ancient technique, described by Aelian (c. 230 A.D.) in his *De Natura Animalium*, involves reaching below a river undercut, groping blindly for a trout and, finding one, stroking its belly until it falls into a sort of trance and can be hauled out. "Trout tickling" was familiar enough in early modern Europe that Shakespeare could use it as a metaphor to describe the hapless Malvolio in *Twelfth Night*: "… here comes the trout that must be caught with tickling" (Act II, Scene 5). (The reader who finds this incredible should check out one of the dozens of trout tickling videos on YouTube.)

According to Ulanski, ancient Egyptians were among the first fly fishers, "as evidenced by a 1400 B.C. temple drawing showing a man holding a short rod to which is affixed seven individual lines, each with a flying insect."[1] Aelian, in his *De Natura Animalium*, wrote not only about tickling trout but also taking them with artificial flies.

But the first detailed discussion in English of fly fishing, in what is also one of the first great how-to manuals, is "*A Treatise of Fyshynge Wyth an Angle*," written by Dame Juliana Berners around 1420 and later published in the *Book of St. Albans* (1496). Dame Juliana gives helpful instructions, with illustrations, in every facet of the sport, including making rods and braiding horse hairs for fishing line. She also is among the first—perhaps *the* first—to place fishing among the "means and causes that lead a man into a happy spirit." "[G]ood sports and honest games are the cause of a man's happy old age and long life. The best, in my simple opinion," declares Dame Juliana, "is fishing, called angling, with a rod and a line and a hook."

The classic on fly fishing as a source of physical and emotional well-being is indisputably *The Compleat Angler*, by Izaak Walton (1653). Walton's book is a primer on fly fishing, but more importantly, it is a celebration of pastoral leisure and the contentment that follows from it, especially for those who take up a fly rod.

> No life, my honest scholar, no life so happy and so pleasant as the life of a well-governed Angler; for when the lawyer is swallowed up with business, and the statesman is preventing or contriving plots, then we sit on cowslip-banks, hear the birds sing, and possess ourselves in as much quietness as these silent silver streams, which we now see glide so quietly by us.

For Walton, fly fishing offers an opportunity for tranquil contemplation and, to use today's terminology, stress reduction. It is "a diverter of sadness, a calmer of unquiet thoughts, a moderator of passions, a procurer of contentedness." And while *The Compleat Angler* is packed with useful observations and instructions for catching fish, the book is remembered today for its lyrical reflections on nature and the contentment that comes from spending time there. Also, it may be the first portrayal of therapeutic fly fishing.

Perhaps fly fishing was an attractive subject for Walton in examining the contemplative life because it is such a rich source of comparisons. Fishing generally has provided us with a treasure trove of metaphors. We fish for compliments; hook a reader; land a contract; hit a snag; net a profit; take someone hook, line, and sinker; bait an antagonist; reel in a sucker; despise bottom-feeders; feel like a fish out of water; suspect something's fishy; prefer to be a big fish in a small pond; go on a fishing expedition; and regret the one that got away—she would've been a real catch—while knowing there are other fish in the sea.

Each cast is a shot at redemption, which is perhaps why fishing is so prominent in the Bible, as in this New Testament introduction to the first disciples:

> And Jesus, walking by the sea of Galilee, saw two brethren, Simon called Peter, and Andrew his brother, casting a net into the sea: for they were fishers. And he saith unto them, Follow me, and I will make you fishers of men. (Matthew, 4:18-19, KJV)

In that most famous of fly-fishing stories, *A River Runs Through It*— the novella by Norman Maclean, but more influentially, the motion picture of the same title—fly fishing is close to religion, thanks to Maclean's memorable scrambling of piety and angling in his book's opening lines:

> In our family, there was no clear line between religion and fly fishing. We lived at the junction of great trout rivers in western Montana, and our father was a Presbyterian minister and a fly fisherman who tied his own flies and taught others. He told us about Christ's disciples being fishermen, and we were left to assume, as my brother and I did, that all first-class fishermen on the

Sea of Galilee were fly fishermen and that John, the favorite, was a dry-fly fisherman.

A River Runs Through It, the movie, not only popularized fly fishing and got a great many people started in the sport, it cemented the bond between fly fishing and spirituality. The angling scenes in the film are incandescent, as when Brad Pitt's character stands on a rock at mid-stream "shadow casting." That iconic moment is captured in the film's publicity poster: the angler in the middle distance and turned away from the viewer with his rod at two o'clock and the fly line frozen in a loopy reverse "Z" high above him like a calligraphy flourish, the figure dwarfed by a wall of trees—a green cathedral with shafts of sunlight slanting down as if through stained glass. This isn't fishing. It's worship.

Maclean is hardly alone in tapping fly fishing as a metaphor for spirituality and self-exploration. "The reason for fishing," writes Ulanski, "is not to find fish but to find oneself—a means to self-discovery and awareness."[2] In much recent non-fiction, fly fishing is depicted as more soul-searching than sport, as in *What the River Knows: An Angler in Midstream*, by Wayne Fields (1990); *Fly Fishing Through the Midlife Crisis*, by Howell Raines (1993); *The Bright Country: A Fisherman's Return to Trout, Wild Water, and Himself*, by Harry Middleton (1993); and *My Life Was This Big: And Other True Fishing Tales*, by Lefty Kreh (2008). Middleton's book is especially relevant here. It is a lyrical meditation on the author's struggle with clinical depression—worsened by his losing a cherished job—and the role fly fishing played in his long recovery.

Today the notion that fly fishing constitutes a search for higher meaning makes unexceptional such titles as *The Spirituality of Fly Fishing: An Introduction* (2016) and *Fly-Fishing—The Sacred Art: Casting a Fly as a Spiritual Practice* (2012). In the first, author Jody Martin truly draws no line between religion and his sport. "To fly fish," he writes, "is to become one with the natural world, to focus all eternity on a single fly and a fish that might rise to it, to feel, through the fly rod, the heartbeat of God." He compares fly fishing to other spiritual practices like prayer and meditation, which he describes as emptying the mind to fill it with God. "And fly fishing quite clearly does both. It empties the mind, and fills it with something else, something pure and unattainable elsewhere." Fly fishing puts us in touch with natural rhythms—insect life cycles, flowing water, the seasons—and then through its own casting rhythms and requirements brings us into harmony with the environment. "I suspect that *everyone* who has fly fished has felt something beyond the stream, something beneath the stones, something more," Martin writes.

The Spirituality of Fly Fishing is a textbook for a beginner's class in fly fishing, and the discussions of spirituality are limited to the introduction and a brief conclusion. These are not merely afterthoughts; however, the book is primarily about fly-fishing basics: gear, casting, knots, and so on. In contrast, *Fly-Fishing—The Sacred Art: Casting a Fly as a Spiritual Practice* is concerned less with the mundane how of fly fishing and more with the religious why.

The co-authors of *Fly-Fishing—The Sacred Art* are Rabbi Eric Eisenkramer and Rev. Michael Attas, a Presbyterian priest and cardiologist. They write in alternating sections as if in an ecumenical dialogue. The first four chapters are organized in the chronology of a day of fishing: getting ready, going to the stream, fishing, and returning home. The final four chapters have to do with fishing with friends (communion), fishing somewhere new, fly tying, and stewardship. Throughout, the authors continually draw parallels between fly fishing and their own religious experiences.

For example, in "Getting There," Eisenkramer compares cars in traffic to trout. "Whether I watch the cars zip by like trout in a stream or get lost in my own thoughts of life and death and memories, no trip to the river is without the potential for reflection." Attas describes his drive to a stream as "sort of a cosmic journey to the heart of our human connection to the Divine, and to all of creation." In "Being There," the rabbi compares retrieving a snagged line or untangling knots to working out spiritual problems, with parishioners or himself. In both instances, it's best to go slow so as not to make matters worse. The murmur of a trout stream reminds the minister, who is also a surgeon, of listening to a patient's heartbeat and the movement of blood through a body. "Blood is, of course, nothing but water with a few extra things thrown in for good measure. Like water, it is the life force of the universe. And so, it is the sound of water that we all come home to when we walk into a river." Attas concludes that when standing in the current, "I sense not separateness from God but union." Eisenkramer is even more explicit, drawing a comparison between wading and immersion in a ritual bath.

> Standing on the trout stream, I remember that the cold waters of the mikvah are called *mayim chaim*, waters of life. Jewish law states that the waters must connect to a natural source, such as collected rainwater. The trout stream is likewise *mayim chaim*, a life-giving place, one that sustains insects and fish, but also replenishes and nourishes the soul of the angler.

In the most intriguing section of *Fly-Fishing—The Sacred Art*, Rev. Attas reflects on early Celtic Christian belief in "thin" or "liminal places," border regions where we can come into contact with God. "These are places," writes Attas, "where we experience the reality of God more purely, more certainly, more radically, more authentically than in other places. And, for me, rivers are often those very thin places." Later in the book, Attas calls rivers "sacred spaces," time on the river "worship," and fly fishing "liturgy, the physical and tangible expression of our shared faith."

For these and other like-minded authors and readers, fly fishing is a spiritual quest. Even if this is the sort of hyperbole Ulanski has in mind, the sentiments are honest and heartfelt, and they resonate. Many find in fly fishing an opportunity for meditation, connection, and personal renewal that they don't find elsewhere. As Martin writes of fly fishing, in what sounds like a passage from a psalm, "It helps me, it restores me, it moves me, it heals me."

Fly fishing heals. Martin presents the connection between fly fishing's spirituality and its power to heal as more or less self-evident. Likewise, many TFF programs speak of this ability almost as a matter of faith. Four Circles Recovery Center says of fly fishing that it is "believed by many to be its own form of therapy," Reeling for Recovery avows "the healing powers of the sport of fly-fishing," and Casting for Recovery presents its retreats as opportunities for women to "experience healing connections with other women and nature."

None of these programs presents fly fishing as magical, nor do they view it in isolation. People struggling with the same challenges clearly benefit a great deal just from coming together and talking about what they are going through with others in the same situation. This is true of combat veterans in TFF programs, as well. The activity of fly fishing unites them with brothers and sisters who have had comparable experiences, speak the same language.

At the same time, fly fishing mends in strikingly personal and individual ways. Thousands of damaged men and women have taken up the sport and art of fly fishing for diversion from sadness and the calming of unquiet thoughts.

Notes

1. Stan Ulanski, *The Science of Fly-Fishing* (Charlottesville: University of Virginia Press, 2003), 2.
2. Ibid, 10.

Part 1.

Therapeutic Fly Fishing for Women with Breast Cancer

Chapter 2

Cast, Mend

A morning with the river muffins

It was calming. I wasn't thinking about my next doctor's appointment or what was going to happen. I was just concentrating on the line and the fish.—Sara

Early on a late-August Sunday, fourteen men in chest waders and fly-fishing vests are chatting idly in small groups in the parking lot of a Dunkin' Donuts in Pulaski, New York. They are an unremarkable sight in this Oswego County village of 2,300 residents, which at one time in its distant past was called, reasonably, Fishville. Pulaski (pull-ASK-aye) is something of a sport fishing mecca, thanks to a sensibly named waterway nearby.

The Salmon River rises in New York State's Tug Hill region, in the foothills of the Adirondack Mountains, and flows 44 miles west through two hydroelectric dams before emptying into Lake Ontario. Each year, the river draws thousands of anglers for the spawning runs of Chinook, Coho, Atlantic salmon, and steelhead. These fish can be monsters. The Great Lakes record Chinook was caught in the Salmon River and weighed nearly forty-eight pounds. That's equal to a small bag of cement mix, if a bag of cement mix could leap out of the water, dance across the surface on its tail, and zing line off a reel. Around this time of year, people in waders and vests line the river on both sides for a chance to hook into one of those behemoths.

But the men standing near their cars outside the Dunkin' Donuts aren't looking forward to a day of fighting big fish, or any fish for that matter. They are Casting for Recovery "river helpers," experienced fly fishers who offer their time and expertise to assist women with breast cancer during their first crack at the sport. They are part of a contingent of volunteers who will gather in about an hour on the river, where they'll be joined by the women on their final day of a two-and-a-half-day retreat.

Today's fishing will take place on the Douglaston Salmon Run, a private, two-and-a-half-mile stretch at the lower end of the river where fish enter from Lake Ontario. Catch-and-release fishing is open to anyone with the cost of admission. The number of anglers on the run at the same time is kept to sixty-five during the early and late parts of the season, and 250 from mid-September through the end of October, when spawning is at its height.

The Douglaston Run is a short drive from the Dunkin' Donuts. Not far in the opposite direction is the Tailwater Lodge in Altmar, where a group of women with breast cancer has spent the weekend on a retreat combining emotional support, health information, and fly-fishing instruction. With lessons in casting and entomology behind them, the women are eager to fish.

The mission of Casting for Recovery is "to enhance the quality of life of women with breast cancer through a unique program that combines breast cancer education and peer support with the therapeutic sport of fly fishing." The guiding principle of the retreats, which are free to participants, is to give the women time away from treatment in a natural setting where they can learn to fly fish while making connections with other women and sharing information about what they are going through.

The program coordinator for Casting for Recovery for Upstate New York is Steve Olufsen, of Rochester, who runs the program along with his mother, Laura. Tall and boyish, Olufsen, 38, has a look true to his last name, with a pale complexion, reddish hair, and a light beard. He has guided anglers on and around Lake Ontario for more than fifteen years. On this morning in Pulaski, Olufsen gets the day started by briefing the river helpers, who form a ragged half-circle in front of him in the parking lot.

"Help the women in and out of the water, even if they say they don't need help. Offer an arm," he says, holding out his own with bent elbow pointed forward as if inviting someone to join him on the dance floor. "Don't grab, and be careful about touching."

Some of the women are recovering from surgeries, Olufsen explains. Some may not be feeling well. Besides, they are inexperienced in wading over slippery stones in moving water. He explains that in case someone takes ill—it happens—a physician will be on hand.

A veteran helper offers a suggestion. "It's good to move the girls around. If one girl catches a fish, you might move someone else there into the hot spot."

Girls? Calling mature women "girls" might in any other context raise eyebrows. But among the river helpers this sort of talk seems less paternalistic than affectionate, even protective. Most of the time they refer to the women as "the ladies." During a previous retreat, one of the participants dubbed the helpers "river muffins," a name that stuck.

With no other suggestions or questions, Olufsen takes the lead in a convoy of cars headed to a section of the Douglaston Run a few miles west of Pulaski. There, in an open field by a tree line, the helpers make final preparations and wait for all-terrain vehicles driven by Douglaston guides to take them to fishing spots on the river. During the wait, one of the helpers, Bruce, reveals that his wife, Sara, is part of today's group.

"She had to be dragged here," he says. "She's not exactly into 'sharing' and therapy. But I think everyone can use some therapy."

Sara was diagnosed with stage 1 breast cancer the previous October.

It was caught early but is an aggressive form of the disease. Not long ago, following surgery, she completed four grueling months of chemotherapy. Bruce hasn't seen her since Friday—spouses are not allowed during the retreat—and today Sara will be paired with a different river helper.

Within the hour, after the men have been driven to their spots in groups of four or five, the women are also transported by ATVs—all-terrain vehicles—to each place, one angler per helper. They are dressed in new waders and spotless fishing vests. There are introductions and a lot of awkward joking.

As one of the women is assisted down a steep cut to the shore, she says, "What's the worst that can happen—I fall on my butt?" She is thin and has pale, papery skin. No hair is visible along the edges of her baseball cap.

The river is wide here but not too wide to throw a stone across, if you throw hard. The far shore is lined with tall grasses, and further inland there are stands of trees spaced far apart. The flat, open ground provides easy movement for anglers looking for a good spot. On this side, the undergrowth of hawthorn, alder, and black elderberry is modestly denser but still offers a view far into the woods. Fly fishers make their way easily along the shoreline and through the trees. Upstream, the river bends gently to the right and out of view.

The water is low but still up to the knees and moving swiftly enough to push a novice off her feet. The helpers follow Olufsen's directions, offering an arm to a dance partner, and the participants take their first tentative steps into the water. Soon the helper/angler pairs are spaced about 10 meters apart at midstream up and down the river.

One of the ladies is worried she'll lose her balance. "It's a little bit slippery," she says. An organizer (except for Olufsen, all are women) stops to take her picture and reassure her that she'll get her stream legs as the day wears on. But she looks uncomfortable casting, as if swing-

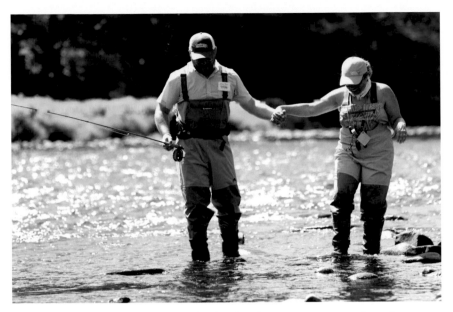

A Casting for Recovery river helper lends a hand to a participant wading the Salmon River. (Courtesy of Casting for Recovery)

ing her arm backward and forward will throw her off her feet, so an assistant brings out a canvas chair, and she spends the morning fishing while seated.

For a half hour or so, not much happens. The sun is beating down out of a cloudless sky. The river is low, the salmon have not moved upstream, and the fishing has been poor for days. Still, a peaceful vibe settles over the groups. The helpers stand behind and to the side of each angler, offering quiet instruction and encouragement.

Brian has his partner using a strike indicator floating eighteen inches above a nymph. When a fish hits the indicator a couple times, Brian wonders aloud if he should switch to a White Wulff—then a fish takes the nymph. There's a flurry of activity as the novice fly fisher tries to keep her line tight, but the fish gets off.

Next, he shows her how, when the fly has reached the end of its drift, to whip her rod low and upstream in a single motion, snapping her wrist as if tossing a Frisbee. This brings the fly to two o'clock and restarts a drift. "Now, mend the line," he says, softly, motioning with his right arm in an upstream bob. She gets the hang of it quickly. Soon she has the line bowed on the water above her fly, allowing it to drift freely and without any drag.

Then there's a subtle shift in the angle of the leader, and the rookie fly fisher raises the rod tip to tighten her trembling line. Fish on! A coordinator on shore shouts and claps, and cheers travel in a steady call and response up and down the river. The first catch of the day is an eight-inch fallfish, whose large silver scales give it the look of a miniature tarpon, which is what locals, with unsubtle irony, call it: the Salmon River Tarpon. Even if it is the largest fish of its kind in this part of the world, the fallfish is still a minnow. But the successful angler holds her catch like a trophy and smiles dazzlingly for photos.

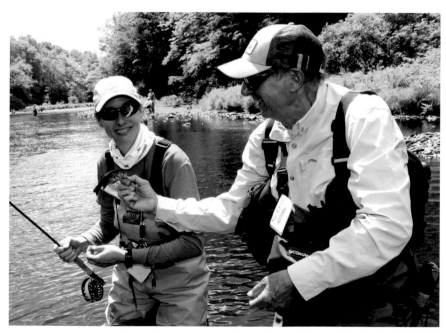

Landing even a tiny fish is a victory for this first-time fly fisher.
(Courtesy of Casting for Recovery)

Not long after this, she catches two more fish; she's learned how to set the hook by snapping the rod heavenward. The other ladies are gaining confidence, as well. One tries out her false cast, but the line usually collapses in a stack in front of her. But she keeps at it. Meanwhile, the helpers are adjusting to the conditions, putting on split-shot to get the flies down to where the fish are hugging the bottom. They are determined to see everyone at least get a fish on.

The temperature rises steadily throughout the morning until it's well into the 80s. Regardless of the heat, the women clearly are enjoying themselves as they focus on casting and mending their lines. The helper/angler pairs become teams and, as many will comment later, friends. And one of the ladies is false casting like a veteran.

At 11:30, the designated quitting time, organizers send out a call for everyone to come in. These shouts are ignored by at least half the pairs, who are working hard to get a fish. It takes a while, but eventually they all make their way reluctantly to shore. The awkwardness with which the morning began has been replaced with an easy familiarity between the men and women. The ladies take hold of their partners' arms and together they wade across the river and back to the riverbank, talking quietly to one another and calling out to the others.

Everyone—river helpers, casting instructors, organizers, medical and psychosocial professionals, local guides, a photographer, a writer, and the ladies—gathers around a half dozen ATVs and two picnic tables in a clearing by the water. There is a lot of bragging and some good-natured regrets about missed opportunities, typical post-fishing chatter.

Throughout the retreat, each of the women has kept a small stone as an emblem of what she was feeling. For many, it represents anxiety or fear. Now they are invited to throw those stones into the Salmon River in a symbolic letting go. A few, not ready yet, slip them into a pocket for another time.

Then it's time for photographs. The final shot is of the ladies with the river in the background, some sitting in a row on the grass, the rest standing behind them holding a Casting for Recovery banner. The composition recalls a team photo from a high school yearbook. Everyone in the picture, including two women whose cancer is terminal, is smiling broadly, as if any moment she will erupt into laughter.

Chapter 3

Why Cast for Recovery?

A surgeon's perspective on therapeutic
fly fishing for women with breast cancer

Cancer… negates the possibility of life outside and beyond itself; it subsumes all living. The daily life of a patient becomes so intensely preoccupied with his or her illness that the world fades away. Every last morsel of energy is spent tending the disease.
—Siddhartha Mukherjee, *The Emperor of All Maladies:*
  A Biography of Cancer

They can't just pick up and go on with their life like it was before.
—Deb Norris

Deb Norris likes to describe herself as a strong North Country woman. In late middle age, she is of medium height and solidly built, with shoulder-length white hair that is less brushed than wind-blown and the ruddy complexion of someone who spends a lot of time outdoors. When she meets a visitor for lunch at a Pulaski restaurant in December, when the temperature is in the 20s, she is wearing a parka over layers of clothing and sturdy winter boots. She talks fast and with her hands—at times she seems to be snatching ideas out of midair—and laughs easily and often.

"I thought I was going to be late," she says, although she's precisely on time. "My tractor wouldn't start this morning, and I've got a cow down." This comes out matter-of-factly, as if she were mentioning an icy windshield.

When Norris isn't attending sick cows on her 89-acre farm in Watertown, N. Y., she's caring for human patients as a board-certified general surgeon with a specialty in breast surgery oncology. She also serves as a medical facilitator for Casting for Recovery and was along for the retreat the past August.

Where farmer Norris is outwardly blasé about an ailing Black Angus, Dr. Norris is passionate when discussing breast cancer. She seems to take personally the damage done to her patients by surgery and post-operative care and to feel responsible for the devastation caused by the treatment of which she is so central a part.

"Some of the things we do to people are pretty gruesome," she says.

Over soup and a sandwich, she describes breast cancer surgery in the sort of detail you usually don't hear in a restaurant. She also uses her hands to mime the surgery in broad gestures.

"You go in there and you cut the breast off of the pectoralis muscle," Norris says. The pectoralis connects the front of the chest with the upper arm and shoulder. "And sometimes you damage it on purpose because the cancer will go through the muscle and into the fascia. So now you've damaged this muscle. Just think of everything you do with your arms and your hands."

She picks up her sandwich with both hands and takes a bite. After she's had a chance to chew, Norris moves on to the next stage of the procedure, removing lymph nodes.

"You pick up the pectoralis muscle with this great big retractor and pull it way over." She reaches across herself with her left hand to imitate grabbing the edge of the table, then pulls up and away as if peeling the lid off a giant Tupperware container. "That exposes your axillary vein, which is a vein this big"—holds up an index finger—"and you cut the fascia off of that and drag that down to two major nerves that give sensation to your hand and movement and, you know, keep you going."

Norris describes all this with a good deal of dark humor born of experience and with professional detachment, and she clearly enjoys the shock value (although when diners nearby seem to be staring at her, she turns down the volume). But through the fabric of her colorful narrative runs a dark thread of guilt.

She says, "Now you've damaged two things for your upper extremities. And just think how important your extremities are. And put on top of that the radiation that does damage to the same structures. And a lot of times when you give people chemotherapy, the nerves are damaged and you get a neuropathy. Even the fine work, they can't do it because of the damage from the neuropathy."

"So now you've damaged major muscles, minor muscles in the upper extremities," Norris says, summing up. "Basically you've made them a cripple."

Norris's guilt comes through more as anger than regret. The care she provides extends and saves lives, but too often it leaves women physically and emotionally ravaged. This is a not uncommon complaint about cancer treatments generally, that the cure can be worse than the disease.

She continues, "First of all, we take off their breast. And in Western society the breast is a big thing. Number two, we take out their ovaries or do something chemically to shut down their ovaries so they're not making estrogen so the cancer doesn't get fed, because most breast cancers are estrogen fed. So now we've taken away their hormones."

To Norris's point, one breast cancer survivor who attended a Casting for Recovery retreat speaks of herself during treatment, which included a double mastectomy, as "not feeling very womanly." "I have no breasts, no hair," she says. "You don't feel yourself, you don't feel very feminine."

But Norris is especially frustrated at the lack of support for women with breast cancer after they have completed treatment, during the long slog back to what can pass for a normal, full life. Her principal gripe is that the women are frequently left to grapple with recovery on their own.

"We've done so many things to them that they can't just pick up and go on with their life like it was before. So many people are isolated."

That isolation is compounded, says Norris, by impediments to some necessary post-surgery therapies. Many breast cancer survivors suffer from lymphedema, chronic swelling in the arms that results from damage to the lymphatic system—the vessels, ducts, and glands (the lymph nodes) that together collect fluid that leaks from blood into tissue throughout the body to feed cells and to gather waste. The collected lymph is transported to glands for filtering and then returned to the circulatory system. Because breast cancer surgery involves removal of lymph nodes, the fluid has nowhere to go, and painful, movement-restricting edema often results. The swelling can be so bad that William Stewart Halsted, a pioneer in breast cancer surgery around the turn of the nineteenth century, called the condition "surgical elephantiasis."[1]

Lymphedema is treatable (although not curable) with doctor-prescribed compression sleeves and garments, or in more severe cases with "complete decongestive therapy": bandaging, draining, and other procedures. It is common to see breast cancer survivors wearing compression sleeves on one or both arms. A sleeve is tighter at the bottom—that is, nearer the hand—than at the top; the graded pressure keeps fluid moving in the right direction.

The compression supplies used in the treatment of lymphedema are medically necessary for the recovery of breast cancer survivors. They help prevent recurrent infections, worsening of the condition, and even disability. They are safe, easy to use, effective—and not covered by many insurance policies.

Insurance companies follow the lead of Medicare, and Medicare does not cover compression treatment supplies because they cannot be classified in any existing benefit category under Medicare law. It is very difficult to state that logic without sarcasm; however, the fault is not Medicare's. This is federal law, and the only body with the authority to change that law by adding or redefining categories is the United States Congress. Now sarcasm is warranted. The Lymphedema Treatment Act, which would mandate coverage of compression treatment supplies, was first introduced in 2010. As of this writing, it remains an active bill in the 2021–2022 Congress.

That the Lymphedema Treatment Act has languished for more than a decade in Washington is, for Deb Norris, symptomatic of a larger problem. Medical care for breast cancer has improved markedly in the past several decades, and women are doing better than ever thanks to aggressive, if debilitating, surgery, chemotherapy, and radiation. But what about the difficult recovery afterward? Medical science does what it can, says Norris, and then sends the women on their way.

"OK, you've completed your treatment, you're cured, go on with your life," she says with mock cheerfulness.

Norris lived with this frustration for years. She thought of her patients in physical therapy, but "going through PT every day is a drag," she says. "And in the hospital you're just in this depressing arena under fluorescent lights." How, she came to ask herself, could she be involved in the recovery of her patients in a happier setting, doing something enjoyable?

The answer came unexpectedly when Norris attended a Breast Cancer Survivorship Conference at The Ohio State University Comprehensive Cancer Center – Arthur G. James Cancer Hospital and Richard J. Solove Research Institute, in 2008. Among the attendees that year were representatives of an organization that provided therapeutic fly-fishing retreats for women with breast cancer.

"I see Casting for Recovery," recalls Norris, "and I think it's the answer to my prayers. I was enthralled. So I got involved that same year. I applied to Casting for Recovery to be a Medical Facilitator, and they said yes."

Notably, Norris was not and is not now a fly fisher. When she learned what Casting for Recovery offered, she saw not so much a day on the water as a novel and engaging form of physical therapy.

"It's the gentle range of motion," she says, abandoning her sandwich to false cast an invisible rod, which fortunately does not gain the attention of a server. "And they can stop when they want to stop. There's no competition. When they learn how to do fly fishing—none of them have before—you get that gentle range of motion. It's stretching the muscles, stretching the scars. Breaking up some of the scars." Too often, Norris says, post-operative breast cancer therapies end too soon. "When people are done with therapy they say, 'Well, that's done,' and they don't do it anymore. And those things that therapy broke up and made better happen again."

We need these extended physical therapies, Norris argues, because cancer survivors are living longer. "That's why these problems are coming to the forefront now," she says. "People never used to have these problems because they'd be dead." Why worry about range of motion in your arm if you don't live long enough to use it?

"If you're fly fishing and you like it and you do it again, maybe with the group you met at Casting for Recovery, and you meet down at the Tailwater and you go out—you're still doing the same thing," says Norris. "So it keeps it constant without having to go to therapy."

Of course, physical rehab is only part of the recovery, maybe not even the most important part, Norris says.

"I don't think you can have anything that severe, whether it's cancer, whether it's traumatic injury from war or a car accident, from a machine, from a farm machine—I don't think you can have something that severe happen to you without it changing you psychologically."

Casting for Recovery retreats also are about peer support, something most women with breast cancer do not seek, according to the organization's surveys. Many women—many people—may be turned off by group therapy and peer support, perhaps viewing these activities as pop-psychology hug-ins. That attitude sets Deb Norris's teeth on edge.

"Some people don't believe in that fluffy, touchy-feely stuff. But Casting for Recovery is different. This is not touchy feely." She punctuates this last statement by stabbing at the air in front of her with an index finger as if pressing an uncooperative button on a vending machine.

"I don't understand why it's looked down on and why it's looked down on in the whole medical community. They've been through a horrible, horrible thing. Why *can't* they cry on someone else's shoulder? Why do we look down on that? What the hell is wrong with *us*?"

Notes

1. S. Mukherjee, *Emperor of all maladies: a biography of cancer.* (Thorndike Press, 2012), 65.

Chapter 4

This Isn't *Bowling* for Recovery

The who, what, and why of a Casting for Recovery retreat

> Snow was just coming down, it's cold, and they're standing in freezing
> cold water, and you could tell that all of them were just enjoying the
> experience. I think they felt powerful.
> —Lisa Green, Casting Instructor

The genesis of *Casting for Recovery*, in 1996, was the root of the connection Deb Norris makes between fly casting and physical therapy for women with breast cancer. The program was the brainchild of a group of women, including Dr. Benita Walton, then a breast cancer reconstructive surgeon (she has since changed her specialty to psychiatry) in Manchester, Vermont. An avid fly fisher, Walton saw in the overhand motion of casting an opportunity for enjoyable, repetitive physical therapy. Also, concerned about her patients' emotional well-being as they and their families faced an uncertain future, Walton proposed to bring women with breast cancer together in a serene natural environment as an assist in the psychic healing process. With the help of medical colleagues, friends, and fellow anglers like professional fly fisher Gwenn Perkins Bogart, along with the support of the Orvis Company, Casting for Recovery got off the ground.

Casting for Recovery foregrounds physical rehabilitation in its literature and on its website when it states that "The gentle, rhythmic motion of fly casting is similar to exercises often prescribed after surgery or radiation to promote soft tissue stretching." But Casting for Recovery retreats go well beyond the physical benefits of fly fishing. "On an emotional level, women are given the opportunity to experience a new activity in a safe environment amongst a supportive group of peers. The retreats provide resources to help address quality of life issues after a breast cancer diagnosis, and a new outlet—fly fishing—as a reprieve from the everyday stresses and challenges of their cancer." The women are brought together "to find inspiration, discover renewed energy for life, and experience healing connections with other women and nature."

Each Casting for Recovery retreat takes place over two-and-a-half days, from Friday afternoon through Sunday. The all-volunteer staff—there are upwards of 1,600 volunteers nationwide—includes at least one medical professional and one psycho–social counselor, as well as several specially trained fly-fishing instructors and a number of river helpers who are paired with the women during their Sunday morning fishing excursion. Organizers take the term "retreat" seriously: This is an opportunity for participants to get away to a place "free of the stresses from medical treatment, home, or workplace." Loved ones are politely but firmly excluded. As the Casting for Recovery website makes clear, participants are encouraged "to step outside of your comfort zone and enjoy a weekend to focus on yourself—in the company of other women who know exactly what you're going through and where you've been. Please leave your husbands, partners and pets at home!" Although breast cancer is not limited to women, men with the disease are not included in the retreats. This is very much a female getaway.

Casting for Recovery offers forty-plus retreats each year for more than 700 women. Each retreat follows the same schedule. After they arrive on Friday afternoon, participants are outfitted with rods, waders, and boots, and directed to their rooms. Later they take part in ice-breaking activities. Saturday is devoted to mini-courses in knot-tying, casting, and stream entomology. Also, the women take part in sessions on medical and psycho-social matters. Finally, on Sunday morning everyone goes fishing for three or four hours. The retreat closes with a luncheon for everyone involved and a graduation ceremony for the women.

A score of volunteers is required for each retreat: a program coordinator to oversee all the arrangements, organize volunteers, and secure tackle and outfits for the women, along with raising money, managing publicity, and attending to myriad details; a participant coordinator to stay in touch with participants and alternates ahead of the retreat; a retreat leader to guide the women throughout the weekend; a medical facilitator; several psycho-social workers; three or four casting instructors; fourteen river helpers; and various others—including retreat alumnae—to help out with whatever is needed. These are packed weekends.

For the event on the Salmon River organized and hosted by Casting for Recovery for Upstate New York, Steve Olufsen (program coordinator) and his mother, Laura (participant coordinator), received forty

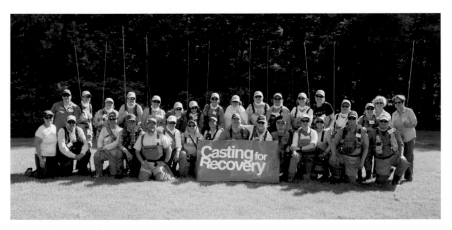

Volunteers and participants gather before heading out to the Salmon River for a morning of fishing. Kneeling to the right of the banner is the author. (Courtesy of Casting for Recovery)

applicants for the fourteen places. Many of the women learned of the retreat from promotional literature Laura, who is a nurse, drops off at cancer clinic waiting rooms around Rochester. She also takes charge of following up with phone calls to selectees and alternates.

"You have to call them frequently and remind them," says Laura. "You feel bad because a lot of them don't recall." The women often suffer from what she calls "chemo brain." These calls are very important. "You just have to get them from point A to point B."

Laura stays busy throughout the weekends. Steve, however, as much as the women appreciate his devotion to the program, has to hang back most of the time.

"My role is a little different because I'm a guy," he says. "Normally the program coordinator would be there for the retreat." So he stays in the background until Sunday morning, when he serves as a river helper.

Olufsen is that rare thing in Casting for Recovery, a man in charge. He learned of the program while attending the annual Lancaster (Pennsylvania) Fly-Fishing Show. Later he contacted the national office to ask about volunteering and found out that the only chapter in New York State was on Long Island, some 400 miles from home.

"So this was an opportunity I saw," says Olufsen. "There's nothing in western New York. It doesn't cost a lot to run one of these programs. What makes me happiest on a personal level is being able to use my talents in any way I can to help people, to inspire people, to give back." Coming from anyone else those words could sound a bit corny, even self-congratulatory. But Steve Olufsen is another too-rare thing: a genuinely selfless, just plain nice guy.

Where Steve is reserved and soft-spoken, his mother is outgoing and bubbly, a hugger. For Laura, the retreats are a time to draw not only on her experience as a nurse but also on a deep well of compassion.

The women know little ahead of time about what will take place over the weekend. (One participant, looking back on her drive to the hotel, says she pictured, and hoped for, a spa treatment.) They aren't exactly kept in the dark, but organizers don't want them to overthink the experience, either. For many, this will be their first time in group discussions about cancer and the first time they will be asked to let their guard down and talk about what they're going through, with the disease and in their personal lives.

"Their marriages break up," Laura says, of several. "It's really very sad."

The moment they arrive, says Laura, "You recognize their personality and the mood. And you can see fear in a lot of them." Some of the women are in the midst of treatment, some are anticipating it, some are long past and adjusting to a life shadowed by cancer. An important job of the organizers is to keep everyone moving.

A regular volunteer casting instructor for Casting for Recovery is Lisa Green, of Rochester, who also works with disabled veterans. She not only teaches the women how to handle a fly rod but mixes with them throughout the weekend, starting from the time they show up on Friday afternoon.

"It's pretty much 'all hands on deck' all weekend," Green says. "We've got equipment that's shipped in on Friday, so we get there Friday about noon to unpack all the waders and the boots and get things set up. Then the women show up and we get them checked in and be sure they know where their rooms are. And then throughout we have all our meals with them and we try to really mix in with them. Because the program is about so much more than the fly fishing."

Green is touching on something central to therapeutic fly-fishing programs of all kinds. Women battling breast cancer, veterans struggling with PTSD, people recovering from drug and alcohol addiction—they all benefit simply from coming together, from being present for one another while doing something new.

The weekend at Casting for Recovery is, says Green, "about the women having a community. And a lot of them have never had any sort of therapy sessions or group counseling, so [what's important is] to get them there and talking to each other—about other things, too—about their experiences with recovery and treatments."

Saturday at a Casting for Recovery retreat is given over to group sessions divided more or less evenly between fly fishing and "quality of life issues" the women are facing. There are two formal sessions on medical issues led by the medical facilitator—Deb Norris in the case of Casting for Recovery for Upstate New York—and other sessions on emotional well-being. These meetings are difficult for the women, in part because they may be reluctant to speak but also because of their empathetic connections to the others. One participant recalls the experience this way: "There were times when I found myself checking out," losing the thread of a discussion after someone had broken down. "I'd wonder what she's feeling right now. I'd wonder if she needs a hug."

The fly-fishing sessions include lessons in tying knots, identifying aquatic insects, and casting. Lisa Green and other instructors take the women outside to practice their casts on the lawn.

"They might have neuropathy in their feet and their hands," Green says, recalling a retreat when the weather turned cold. "We were giving them casting lessons and it was sleeting. And we were just mothering them. And there were no complaints, just huge ear-to-ear grins." That spirit carried over to the fishing on Sunday morning. "Snow was just coming down, it's cold, and they're standing in freezing cold water, and you could tell that all of them were just enjoying the experience. They weren't worried about feeling uncomfortable. I think they felt powerful."

Green finds the separation of responsibilities among the volunteers liberating. "They always have licensed psychotherapists there who can lead counseling sessions. And they always have a medical doctor there.

This is nice for us because we can just focus on fly fishing because we know their other needs are being taken care of."

Another casting instructor, Joanne Hessney, is herself a physician, so she doubles as an informal medical facilitator while teaching the women to handle a fly rod. She describes a "tectonic shift" among oncologists in encouraging cancer patients to live in the moment. The women on the retreat, she says, may be focused, quite understandably, on what will happen next, like chemotherapy. While giving casting instruction, Hessney encourages the women to put those matters out of mind for now. "You don't have to worry about that until you have to worry about that," she recalls saying to them. "Don't dwell on it."

Hessney sees fly fishing as perfect for making someone focus on the present because its novelty requires concentration and focus to accomplish something gratifying and fun.

"Can you think of a more foreign activity?" Hessney asks. "This isn't *Bowling* for Recovery. It's extra foreign. There's no way they can spend the day learning about fly fishing and still worry about chemo."

Of their morning on the Salmon River, Green says, "I can see when the women are out on the river and fishing they're not thinking, 'I'm a sick person' or 'I've got to go to treatment.' They're thinking about what they're doing and whether they're wading safely. It's that focus for them that I think is such a stress release."

Green, who like many of those involved in Casting for Recovery, is passionate about fly fishing, extols the therapeutic benefits of the natural setting. "You feel connected to nature in such an intense way," she says. "You're really immersed in nature, and to me that's special. One of the things is the sound of the water. It's such a soothing thing when you hear that. And the rhythm of casting—there's something about that, too, that rocking motion that is soothing."

As therapy, fly fishing has a lot going for it: relaxation, focus, achievement, exercise, and the restorative effects of nature. That getting out-

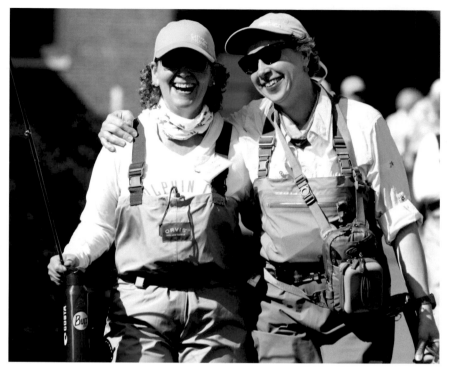

Women on Casting for Recovery retreats often form lasting bonds.
(Courtesy of Casting for Recovery)

doors into natural environments is good for us is not only conventional wisdom but established science. In fact, the stretch of the Salmon River where Casting for Recovery takes the ladies is, as we shall see, a nearly textbook illustration of current theory on natural spaces conducive to human well-being.

The community the women enjoy on these weekends also is critical to the healing that takes place. One participant, Leslie, says of her experience on a retreat, "I got new sisters. I feel like if I'm ever depressed or feeling bad I have someone I can call who really understands what I've been through, what I'm going through."

Nevertheless, for the majority of the women, Casting for Recovery amounts to a single weekend—a memorable one to be sure, but still two-and-a-half days in a life that has been upended. Many of the participants may never pick up a fly rod again. Regardless, although Steve Olufsen would be delighted to see the women become fly fishers, he knows the Casting for Recovery experience changes lives.

"They've tried something new," he says. "Maybe they knew what fly fishing was and always wanted to try it. It's something new to them. Maybe they don't want to continue with it. But maybe they'll go on and try something else that's new. They had fun, and maybe they didn't know they could have fun until this point in time. So now they're going to try having fun doing something else—maybe it's hiking, maybe it's some other activity. That realization can happen at that retreat."

The women discover many things about themselves during these weekends. They speak movingly and vividly of their experiences, often forging links between their inner lives and fly fishing, between the journey of recovery and the course of a river. Sometimes these metaphors are prompted by program volunteers; more often they arise spontaneously. Something about fly fishing in crystalline waters flowing through a lovely natural setting seems to inspire these figurative connections.

It's best to allow the women of Casting for Recovery to describe their experiences in their own words. First, however, we consider how metaphors are used at a Casting for Recovery retreat and how each woman's unique response to those metaphors reminds us of her individuality, which can get lost in all the talk of cancer and its effects. That discussion leads to a related topic, how cancer itself has been employed as a metaphor and what that usage tells us about how we imagine and respond to the disease. In all these connections, there is a lesson. It teaches us how we, the healthy, should face and listen to the unwell.

Chapter 5

In the Bad Rapids

Metaphors of fly fishing and cancer

Illness is the night-side of life, a more onerous citizenship. Everyone who is born holds dual citizenship, in the kingdom of the well and in the kingdom of the sick. Although we all prefer to use only the good passport, sooner or later each of us is obliged, at least for a spell, to identify ourselves as citizens of that other place.
—Susan Sontag, *Illness As Metaphor*

Fly-fishing therapies of all kinds mine angling's rich vein of metaphors for emblems of seeking, persistence, and redemption. The river itself, where the fly fisher stands at midstream, searching, is a ready symbol of a life, with its mysterious sources, loopy meanders, chaotic rapids, smooth runs, dark pools, and abruptly reversing eddies.

Casting for Recovery—a name with almost Biblical, redemptive echoes—takes advantage of these metaphors in an ice-breaking exercise on the first night of each retreat, when the organizers begin building a community of breast cancer survivors. The women learn the different parts of a trout stream—marked on the floor with small signs: run, riffle, eddy, rapids, pool—and are asked to stand in the section that matches their emotional state and talk about what they're going through. For many of the women, this is the first time they have spoken about feelings they've kept buried.

"It's amazing how the different parts of the stream can bond to their emotions," Laura Olufsen says. "They very quickly recognize the fact that they all have something in common, and they open up."

Sara, who we met earlier, chose the turbulence-free run as a metaphor for where she is in her recovery. With surgery and chemo behind her and with life returning to something like normal, she says, "I'm feeling really calm and looking for ways to keep myself centered."

But, no surprise, many of the women place themselves in the rapids. They see their lives as in turmoil and out of their control, with cancer always there to knock them off their feet.

Curiously, one of the participants, Katie, who was well past treatment, *wanted* to be in the rapids. "It was like a higher risk area in the stream," she says. "I felt probably healthier so I was braver. I placed myself in the area where there was more risk involved."

These contrasting responses to the mock trout stream activity are a reminder that, while these women have breast cancer in common, they remain individuals with unique personalities and distinctive lives. For those who are well, this is easy to lose sight of when cancer becomes someone's defining characteristic. Gilda Radner, while struggling for three years with the ovarian cancer that finally took her life, would introduce herself as "the person who used to be Gilda Radner." Perhaps she wanted to remind everyone, with the sort of offbeat humor she was famous for, that a cancer survivor should never be mistaken for a collection of symptoms and survival rates.

This is a challenge for all of us. We come face to face with it when we run into someone we know well who recently has been diagnosed. What's the right thing to say? What subjects should we avoid? *Should* we be avoiding anything or is it best just to confront the subject head on? The very particularity of breast cancer's manifestation in a woman and the facts of her novel experience and singular identity despite the illness are at the heart of Casting for Recovery.

The women who come to the retreats struggle with this as well. Some are reluctant to talk about the disease and would just as soon not be thought of as citizens of the kingdom of the sick. Others are like Reina, who when out in public practically challenged strangers to look away from her bald head, which she not only refused to cover but adorned with a henna tattoo.

"Here I am," she seemed to be saying. "I'm still me."

Those of us among the well are no good at talking about cancer any more than we are comfortable talking about death, as if our silence might keep these feared conditions—one potentially lethal, the other, well, certainly—at bay. We have scores of euphemisms for death, many of them in the sort of humorous vein ("assumed room temperature," "took a dirt nap") that can seem like attempts at cheerfulness in the face of something terrifying, like whistling past the graveyard. Of course, except in fiction, we don't have awkward conversations with the dead about their situations. With cancer survivors, on the other hand, our interactions are fraught and uncomfortable, in large part because our own healthiness is an embarrassment. We struggle to find the right words.

It is a remarkable fact that until fairly recently in the history of cancer treatment, even medical professionals were reluctant to speak candidly to patients about their cancers, not out of squeamishness but for fear the subject would be needlessly upsetting. Writing in the late 1970s, Susan Sontag described how at that time in France and Italy, "It is still the rule for doctors to communicate a cancer diagnosis to the patient's family but not to the patient; doctors consider that the truth will be intolerable to all but exceptionally mature and intelligent patients."

As recently as 1993, an article in the *Journal of Clinical Oncology* could begin, "Continuing controversy surrounds the extent to which patients should be informed of their diagnosis and its implications."[1] Imagine: a controversy just a few decades ago over whether to be honest with a cancer patient about a disease that could kill her. The authors of "Cancer by another name: a randomized trial of the effects of euphemism and uncertainty in communicating with cancer patients" tested assumptions about the use of euphemisms (specifically, "illness" instead of "cancer") when communicating with cancer patients. The authors wanted to know if speaking explicitly and directly to patients about their disease—at the time, not the norm—caused greater anxiety than employing euphemisms and indirection. They learned that ambiguity "appeared to distort the reality of cancer for these patients and resulted in poorer reported adjustment." Further, their findings "suggest that cancer patients might be highly susceptible to any implication that cancer is confusing and frightening to the extent that even doctors or nurses cannot discuss it openly. Conversely, if health professionals are frank and unambiguous in the words they use, cancer will continue to evoke anxiety in the short-term, but patients will feel more capable of coping with it."[2] In other words, candor hurts initially, like ripping off a bandage. But the patient is better off for the honesty in the long run. "More talk about cancer," the study authors conclude, "might help to reduce the fear and shame."[3] They are referring to those emotions in cancer survivors; however, they could just as easily mean all of us.

All this is to say that cancer is a singularly dreaded disease. In *Illness as Metaphor*, Sontag writes that in the not-so-distant past, tuberculosis was the most feared illness. "Now it is cancer's turn to be the disease that doesn't knock before it enters, cancer that fills the role of an illness experienced as a ruthless, secret invasion...." Sontag argues that when a disease is mysterious and terrifying, when it is more dreaded than understood, we are apt to use that illness as a metaphor for whatever we fear most.

She writes, "Any important disease whose causality is murky, and for which treatment is ineffectual, tends to be awash in significance. First, the subjects of deepest dread (corruption, decay, pollution, anomie, weakness) are identified with the disease. The disease itself becomes a metaphor.

"Feelings of evil are projected onto a disease," argues Sontag. "And the disease (so enriched with meanings) is projected onto the world."

It is crucial to emphasize here that what Sontag has in mind is unlike TFF programs' use of metaphors. Casting for Recovery links fly fishing and trout streams to the interior lives of cancer survivors. These are metaphors for emotions and renewal.

In contrast, Sontag, who herself battled cancer for many years and ultimately succumbed to it, writes out of anger. She asserts that cancer has become a metaphor for evil. We see what she had in mind when we recall one of the most famous figurative uses of the illness.

John Dean, White House counsel to President Richard Nixon from 1970 to 1973, testified before the Senate Watergate Committee (June 1973) that he had discussed the Watergate break-in and subsequent cover-up with Nixon in the Oval Office.

"I began by telling the president that there was a cancer growing on the presidency and that if the cancer was not removed the president himself would be killed by it," Dean said. The consequences of the immoral and illegal activities undertaken by Nixon and those loyal to him were, like a cancer, growing out of control and would, if not "removed," bring about the death of Nixon's presidency.

Investing an illness with meaning in this way, linking it with evil, makes the disease all that more difficult to discuss truthfully. Better to turn away, to avoid it. Worse, using cancer as a metaphor for out-of-control wickedness cannot help but reflect on cancer survivors. "The people who have the real disease are… hardly helped by hearing their disease's name constantly being dropped as the epitome of evil," Sontag writes. Cancer as metaphor is yet another cruelty.

"My point," writes Sontag, "is that illness is *not* a metaphor, and that the most truthful way of regarding illness—and the healthiest way of being ill—is one most purified of, most resistant to, metaphoric thinking."

We must, in other words, strip cancer of its mysteries and malevolent associations and commit to facing it head on. We must look directly into the faces of those with the disease and listen closely to their stories.

Notes

1. S. M., Patterson, P. U. Patterson, P.N. Butow, H.H. Smartt, W.H. Mccarthy and M.H. Tattersall, M. H. (1993). Cancer by another name: a randomized trial of the effects of euphemism and uncertainty in communicating with cancer patients. *Journal of Clinical Oncology, 11*(5), 989996. doi:10.1200/jco.1993.11.5.989, 989.
2. Dunn et al., 995.
3. Dunn et al., 996.

Chapter 6

The Voices of Casting for Recovery

*Five women speak about breast cancer,
fly fishing, and hope*

Sara

A week after the Casting for Recovery retreat, Sara sits on the deck behind her home in western New York on a sparkling late-summer day. She is petite and pretty. Dressed in blue jeans and sneakers, Sara, who is 48, has the fresh-faced look of a younger woman. She lost her shoulder-length hair during chemo, but now it's growing back in dark curls, which peek out from under her baseball cap. "I *loved* my hair," she says.

"Bruce [her husband] signed me up for the fly-fishing retreat behind my back," she says, laughing. Reserved and self-effacing, Sara was reluctant to take part in group discussions. "But I decided I'd try it for him."

She admits to some guilt, as though her own experience somehow did not measure up to what others were going through. It didn't help that she traveled to the retreat and roomed with a woman whose breast cancer had metastasized and was in its final stages.

The retreat was often emotional, Sara recalls, particularly when women discussed recurrences of their cancer. These were her least favorite moments. The make-believe trout stream icebreaker, however, helped her locate herself on the journey from diagnosis to recovery and health.

Sara recalled this activity as "a great way to sneak in talking about *things* but also involved fishing and learning about different types of water." She placed herself in the run. "I'm still plugging along, still have obstacles and going through things. But I'm not where I was. I was going through surgeries, and there was some chaos in my family. Now I'm feeling really calm and looking for ways to keep myself centered."

The ladies chose spots all along the stream's changeable course, but many planted themselves in the rapids.

"My heart just ached for some of these women," Sara says.

She came to the retreat after two decades of marriage to a fly fisherman whose passion for the sport she did not share.

"Going through my life and having three kids, I thought of fly fishing as my enemy because Bruce would leave and go fishing." She pictured the sport as little more than "standing in a stream with bugs."

Besides, Sara recalls imagining fly fishing as complicated and probably stressful, and more stress was the last thing she needed.

"When something happens to you like this, you wonder, well, what else can happen? You go through a lot of panic. The past couple years of my life have been traumatic for me. So you're always on guard about what else can happen. All of a sudden you're worried about everything and everyone."

That morning in August when she arrived at the Douglaston Run, the only thing on Sara's mind was trying out her new casting skills.

"I was excited. All that practice casting—I wanted to try it out. And it was such a beautiful day and a beautiful place."

And quiet: For Sara and everyone else the day started slowly. It took the river helpers a while to figure out where those few fish were—hugging the bottom—and how to get a fly on top of them. This left long stretches of time for thinking. But about what?

"I wasn't thinking about anything but fishing," says Sara. "It was calming. I wasn't thinking about my next doctor's appointment or what was going to happen. I was just concentrating on the line and the fish. That's all I was focusing on. It was a great escape."

She was rooted solidly in a tranquil, forgetful present: "I really did forget I had cancer."

She recalls, "It's such a sensory experience in every way. The sun and the scenery and the sound of the water and the cold of the water. It's such a great—being in the moment. You're so focused and concentrating, and then you catch a fish! It's the rush of it."

About fly fishing, Sara says she "gets it now." She's even changed her mind about the insects. After the short course on entomology, she looks forward to standing in a stream in a mayfly hatch or spinner fall, amid a blizzard of bugs.

"I think I changed after the retreat," Sara says. "During this whole time of being sick and so tired all the time, and 'Woe is me,' I realized what a great feeling that was doing something outside my comfort zone. Now I'm feeling like I have to search out other ways and do more of that."

Sara hadn't felt like this since she got sick. She thinks about her roommate on the retreat, whose cancer now is terminal. She told Sara she wants to try everything she can while she can.

"One thing I learned from this experience from the other women: They are living in the now, *really* living in the now. They don't know how much time they have. I'm not going to wait until some time when that happens to me. *I'm* living in the now."

"I seem to have calmed down. I'm realizing how important it is to be happy."

The final morning of the retreat, when the fishing was done and the ladies were invited to throw their stones—those personal totems—into the Salmon River, Sara realized she had left hers in a sweatshirt in a car. She and Bruce are already making plans for a fly-fishing trip when she'll have a chance to cast the stone away. Her destination choice is Florida, where she can stand on a beach, rear back, and fling her burden into the ocean.

Reina

In her favorite photograph, Reina is resting her head on the shoulder of her teenaged daughter, who has turned to kiss her mother on her bald crown. Reina is smiling faintly and her eyes are closed as if she were asleep. The photo was taken three years ago when she was in the midst of four-and-a-half months of chemotherapy, followed by seven weeks of radiation.

Reina, 52, attended the Casting for Recovery of Upstate New York retreat in fall 2015. She was an alternate and was at work when she got the phone call, on the very Friday the retreat began, telling her a spot had opened at the last minute when someone dropped out. Today, sitting in a conference room near her office in Rochester, she recalls that moment.

"I told my boss, 'I'm leaving.'" Reina has large eyes and a no-nonsense personality. Before she got sick, she was an avid weightlifter. Her manager didn't try to stop her.

"I found it very emotional," says Reina. "Part of me, I went there going, 'I got a raw deal. This really kinda sucks. I got two primary cancers.'" Tests following her breast cancer diagnosis revealed she also had ovarian cancer. "And I was also really, really grateful I got breast cancer because that's how I found out about the ovarian cancer."

That was two years before the day she left work to travel to Pulaski for the Casting for Recovery retreat. Getting that last-minute phone call, being jolted out of her Friday routine, was not unwelcome, but it did snap into focus what Reina tries daily to keep in the blurred background. "You almost relive your diagnosis again."

"The thing a lot of cancer survivors won't tell you," Reina says, "is you see it every day you look in the mirror. Every day you look in the mirror you see your scars. I put the part where you're going to die behind me. 'I've got two cancers, I'm going to die—this really sucks.' But there's always that thought in the back of your head: it can reoccur, it can reoccur."

After she arrived at the Casting for Recovery retreat, Reina took part in the mock-stream icebreaker. "I was in the bad rapids," she says. "Everything is going so fast. Even two years later. Even three years later. There's a lot of turmoil, a lot of worry. I didn't think I was in the rapids, but being there forced me to see that, 'Yeah, you're still in the rapids.'"

Once she settled in, though, Reina was happy to be among other cancer survivors. She found solace and strength, not so much in what she received, but in finding herself in a position to help the women she met. She was energized by the opportunity to be important to others.

"What helped me was I was able to step outside of myself and worry about the others," says Reina. "I was able to help some of them. When you're sick, you start asking yourself, 'What value do I have for anyone else?' You're just taking from everyone. I wasn't giving anything back. Being at the retreat made me feel back to who I was before. I was self-sufficient, a doer, not a taker. It was nice to go there and give back to someone."

She was also in a place where volunteers like Joanne Hessney and Lisa Green worked hard to keep her from dwelling on cancer. "They truly wanted to do something to help you get out of your own mind for a while," says Reina. "There are times on the retreat when you're thinking about [cancer]. But when you're on the river fly fishing: I'm trying to figure out how to cast and when that fish is going to come by, and I'm trying to figure out how to read the water. I don't have time to be thinking about anything else but that. And then I start thinking it's so nice out here, and it's a beautiful day, and the fresh air."

Reina's recollection of her day on the water is a stunning mix of images and emotions, like notes for a poem. She experienced fly fishing as if she were living inside a metaphor linking the flowing river and chemotherapy, a metaphor that was transformed into chemo's reverse, a physical and psychic cleansing.

She says, "I was just as nervous that day going into the river as I was the first day of chemo. Those two days melded together. I was worried, what's going to happen, how am I going to feel? I'm concerned if I'll fall and break something. How's it going to feel? And that's how I felt about chemo. So those two days were sort of merging together in that particular moment."

The ordeal of chemotherapy is a constant presence in Reina's life. Memories of the treatment are reawakened by smells and sights, and abruptly she finds herself reliving the trauma, a phenomenon characteristic of Post-Traumatic Stress Disorder (PTSD). Talking about these moments, as when she recalled the day she got the phone call at work inviting her to the retreat, she can sound like a reluctant time traveler who is continually and without warning plucked from the present and transported to a disturbing past. This is what happened initially on the morning she arrived at the Salmon River to meet the river helpers and try out her new skills with a fly rod. But the experience morphed into something fantastic. She recalls the moment in a kind of ecstasy, here and there punctuating her narrative with exclamations and shouts.

"I'm here but, gosh, I feel like I'm sitting all over again for chemo. Slowly, the vision of the hospital and the drip goes away because the stream is the drip of the chemo—for me—and I realize—whope! No, this is water that *I'm* in! It's not coming into me! It was sort of neat. Wow, this is really good! I'm not getting poisoned, I'm kind of going in and I'm relaxing. This was time when I felt so good. I hadn't felt so good and so relaxed in a long time. I wish I could wake up every day and look forward to something like this. And I felt everything is going to be OK. I don't need to worry about my next chemo session or my next radiation—because once you get in the water...."

It is impossible not to see Reina's experience as a kind of baptism, although there is nothing overtly religious in her description of that morning. In the Christian tradition, baptism is an immersion in water symbolizing purification but also regeneration, renewal. Her account also brings to mind Rabbi Eisenkramer's associating fly fishing with a ritual bath: "Standing on the trout stream, I remember that the cold waters of the mikvah are called *mayim chaim*, waters of life."

Regardless, something profound happened to Reina on the river that had less to do with catching fish than with being outdoors and standing in flowing water.

"I remember closing my eyes and thinking, things are just getting washed out of you. All the poisonous chemo in me is getting away. It wasn't about the cancer leaving me, oddly enough. It was about the treatment leaving me. I could visualize things just leaving my body."

Reina, like others who have been through chemotherapy, is quick to point out that it was the treatment rather than the cancer that made her feel so sick. But that morning on the river "kind of took that all away," she says. "I didn't want the day to end. I can still remember how it smelled. I remember the smell of the waders. The smells sort of erased the smells and tastes related to chemo. It was one of the best days of my life."

Like every woman who attends a Casting for Recovery retreat, Reina was given a stone to keep with her throughout the weekend. Hers was smooth and flat, perfect for rubbing.

"I'm a rubber of things—that was perfect. I worry a lot. That stone was a nice way to release all the things I was worrying about. And as I was rubbing, it was a way to transfer all my thoughts into the stone."

After her transformative experience on the river, Reina was ready to let her stone go.

"Probably for the first time since I had cancer, I was able to let go of some of the things, not all of them. Some of the stuff I was able to really let go."

She recalls actually feeling lighter after throwing her stone into the Salmon River.

"I thought, 'You know, I don't have to worry about this part anymore.'"

Katie

Katie talks about her experiences with breast cancer and with Casting for Recovery over coffee in a crowded Starbucks. She is in late middle age, thin and fit, a life-long outdoorswoman. Frequently as she speaks, her voice becomes husky and tears well up in her eyes, which she dabs at with a crumpled tissue. Her raw emotions are never far from the surface.

"I did cancer in 2013," she says. "It robbed me of 2013."

Katie talks as if now she could will cancer out of her life. She is pained at the suggestion, which she's heard many times, that she will "always be a cancer victim."

"I'm sort of an anti-peg-me-as-a-cancer-person. I don't want to be among the sick. I want to be among the healthy."

Two years after her treatment, she heard about Casting for Recovery but was ambivalent about taking part. The way she saw it, she was "totally done with cancer. I'm just like a regular person now."

What she was really interested in, she says, was adding another outdoor activity to her growing list of favorites: hunting, kayaking, surfing, snowboarding. "I didn't want to be in a cancer group," she says. "I just wanted to learn to fly fish."

So, Katie applied, was accepted, and attended the 2015 Casting for Recovery retreat on the Salmon River. From the start, she held herself back emotionally. But as the weekend unfolded, she gradually, grudgingly, let down her guard.

"Laura called to ask if I would be willing to take someone in my car. I'm not really a girlfriend kind of person. But you have to do this. You have to be a human being and get out of your comfort zone and bless other people."

Nevertheless, Katie kept her distance after they arrived at the Tailwater Lodge. "I tried my best not to participate other than learning how to fly fish."

She was even tentative during the mock-stream icebreaker, placing herself in calm water.

"It was something about being in a comfort zone but willing to go out just a little bit."

When the ladies went fishing that October, it was very cold and a light snow was falling. These conditions were nothing new for Katie, though.

"I hunt, too, so I had clothes and I knew how to bundle up and be warm." She felt very much in her element. "I have always been a water person, and I felt healing when I got by water. Even when I went through treatment I had to go to the lake and just see water." The Salmon River had a similar effect on Katie. Like her peer on that retreat, Reina, she saw and felt metaphorical connections between the rushing water and her recovery.

"When you can look out and see the power of it and see how it gets through things and around things, and a tree gets down it still goes around it, I really can relate to that. The fact that obstacles get in its way and it goes around them to where it's going anyway, we kind of have to be that strong." The challenges of cancer and treatment were transformed into "branches, tree roots, rocks."

For all her self-reliance and will to best cancer, Katie recognizes she has not been alone in facing the disease. She talks gratefully of how her boyfriend cared for her throughout chemotherapy and how her children came home from college, against Katie's wishes, to comfort and help her.

At the time, she thought, "I'm okay. I don't need anyone's help." She came to realize, though, that the current she found herself in was swift and often treacherous. "And I think that's the stream, too. You know you can't be out there by yourself." That surrender to illness was difficult for Katie.

"Today, every year, I always think I'm so much healthier. But another year goes by and I think, 'Oh, my God, I wasn't that healthy. Not as healthy as I am now.'"

She thinks making concessions to cancer and accepting help are especially hard for mothers. "They've been strong for their families and now they can't be."

Wading in the stream with a river helper, the women can regain a sense of control and even victory. They come up against the other-ness of fly fishing in a place they've never been—Katie had only walked across shallow streams before when hunting—and find they are up to the challenge.

Katie says, "It's definitely beyond their reach; they're out of their element. A big thing about fly fishing is it's so different from anything those people would do. So different. Women learning about bugs. And I think that's a big thing of it. There was a seriousness about fly fishing."

Katie had tried another cancer support group. "I went to a sewing group. But sewing and knitting—it keeps you in that victim or damaged mode, because it's a gentle thing to do. And after all," she says, sarcastically, "we have cancer. Where this [fly fishing] is like we're going to go out and conquer the world because we just survived cancer."

She went to Casting for Recovery to learn to fly fish; at least that's what Katie told herself. When the fishing was done, though, she had found her old self.

"I surfed, I snowboarded. I was always out there risking a broken bone. I'm ready to be out there again. I think I got cautious with the cancer. A lot of us just want to reach for the stars now. Why are we doing anything less than the ultimate of what we can do? Because life is short, and it's terminal for all of us."

"I always had long hair, and losing it was hard," Katie says, reflecting on her time during treatment. "I don't think you can say that among healthy people because they want you to be thankful that the cancer's over. And you are. But you still want to be 100 percent back to who you were. And your hair is part of your identity. That's a big thing to get around emotionally. None of us should be vain."

Katie says her son told her cancer was a cure for vanity. "And it does cure some vanity issues, and the worth of things vs. people, or your health. You get a different perspective. It's hard to tolerate typical people, because they're just not getting it." She is constantly reminding herself, "Stop worrying about things. Stop worshipping *things*."

Looking back on the retreat, Katie says, "I didn't see it coming that I would get emotional. I didn't see it coming. I got so emotionally healed that when I got back, people actually said I was different My friends *knew* I was different. It is that crossing over a bridge. It put things behind us in a really healthy way. One girl, she found God. She was so touched. She turned her life around."

"When I got back, I called Steve and said, 'OK, I'm a part of this. You're stuck with me.'"

Katie became a "participant coordinator" and now assists at retreats as an alumna. She looks forward to encouraging other women to see fly fishing as a means of pushing beyond what they think they're capable of and resetting their lives. When she returned to Pulaski as a participant coordinator for a retreat, she took part in the icebreaking exercise again. Where she was unsure of herself the year before, settling for a calm place in the water, now she sought out "a higher risk area in the stream. I felt probably healthier so I was braver." She planted herself boldly in a place "where there was more risk involved."

Katie once was reluctant even to talk with others about cancer. Now she is committed to helping other breast cancer survivors by introducing them to fly fishing at Casting for Recovery retreats. She carries with her a card she received from a participant, and now she brings it out to read its message aloud: "'You were right, it's life changing.'"

Leslie

"At first, I thought it was kind of strange because here I am going through chemo, radiation and not feeling very womanly, you know, had a double mastectomy, and I thought this program was like a spa. You don't feel yourself, you don't feel very feminine. And I want to get pampered. I want to go somewhere and get a manicure and a pedicure, a facial. You know, feel more womanly. But no—we're going fly fishing!"

Leslie is a young African-American woman, in her thirties, with an attitude and a loud laugh. When she feels the need to correct someone, she shouts, "Hell-OH!" During the Casting for Recovery retreat she attended in 2015, everyone called her Trouble.

"I don't like to see people down," she says. "I don't like to see people depressed. That's how I got the name Trouble. I was always laughing and making jokes."

Leslie's rowdy good humor has been challenged the past few years since being diagnosed, in 2014, with stage 3 breast cancer. Today, chatting over coffee in a Rochester diner, she mentions, almost as an afterthought, that her cancer has returned and she is once again in treatment.

"I feel like I've been through a war. And I have: I have war wounds and I have PTSD. Now sometimes when I go to the doctor I start shaking because I've gone through so much. What are they going to take from me now? They've taken everything."

There's more: "I lost two friends to breast cancer. A year ago, I lost a friend while I was going through treatment. You feel that survivor remorse because she died, and I didn't. Like people who were on a plane that crashed when there are survivors but others die."

Still, she says, "I'm proud of being a survivor. Cancer's not the end all, be all. You have to enjoy life. We could get hit by a car walking outside. You gotta take it for what it is."

Leslie went to the retreat not knowing what to expect and not feeling especially enthusiastic.

"I was thinking I wasn't going to have a good time. This was just a way to get away for a little bit."

But once she got to Pulaski and met the other women, Leslie quickly became aware of how few opportunities she had had to open up about her experiences with cancer.

"I was *very* eager to talk about it," she says. "It's hard to put into words what you're going through. And it's so helpful for others that are going through the same thing. It's hard to talk with someone who hasn't gone through it. It's frustrating sometimes."

That frustration extended into her medical care, as well. She often felt a total loss of control, a helplessness that is at odds with her in-your-face personality.

"Doctors are used to being right. And you can be intimidated. They are smarter than me. They've been in school probably longer than I've been alive."

The medical sessions at Casting for Recovery were a revelation for Leslie. For the first time since she learned she was sick, she had a chance to talk openly and unhurriedly about how cancer was reshaping her life, especially her life as a woman.

"I was excited because there was a doctor there who we got to talk to and ask questions. And she was awesome. I felt in more of a relaxed atmosphere than in a doctor's office where it's kind of cold and you're feeling insecure. But this was an environment where you can feel relaxed, you're among people who've been through the same things you have. It felt like I was talking to a friend rather than a doctor. She was patient, and she was understanding, and she was concerned. She stayed the night and she told us we could come to her in the middle of the night if we had questions."

The fly-fishing sessions were more of a challenge for Leslie. She gives the impression that she was the class clown, Trouble for instructors. And handling a fly rod did not come naturally to her.

"They taught you how to hold the rod and cast it," says Leslie. "Oh, my god, I must have been in the remedial class because I could not get it!"

Her casting instructor taught her to mime holding a telephone to her ear and then offering it to someone else. Making a casting motion with one hand, Leslie says, "Pick up the phone"—hand to the ear—"it's for you"—hand thrust forward—"pick up the phone, it's for you. That worked for me. I could get that. I'm used to picking up the phone."

These initial difficulties with a fly rod notwithstanding, Leslie was enjoying herself.

She says, "We were a lively group. We were fun, we were like family. We got along great with each other. We were loud and rowdy and having a good time."

This spirit carried over to the group's morning on the Salmon River. Good thing, too, because it snowed. Leslie took the situation as another opportunity to lighten the mood.

"We're going in the water and I've got this walking stick. And I held it up like Moses and said, 'We're going to separate this water!'"

But wasn't she led in by a river helper?

"He was a river *muffin*! Hell-OH!" Leslie takes credit for coming up with the name. "We had all been through a lot. We weren't feeling womanly or attractive. A lot of us had serious side effects. The men there made us feel great. They made us feel like a woman, they made us feel comfortable. They weren't at all apprehensive about our treatment."

No outdoorswoman, Leslie was apprehensive about the fishing. She had never waded in a river before.

"At first I was like—we're going to be out there for a whole hour?

Three hours? What? I'm not going to be doing this for three hours! But once we got out there, we were having such a good time. We were having a competition. And we had the river muffins. Time just flew by. And it was snowing while we were on the river, and that made it even more awesome."

Remarkably, given her struggles, Leslie caught the first fish that day. But this seems only incidental to her, hardly worth mentioning. What she recalls most vividly is standing at midstream on a day when many people would prefer to be by a fire.

"It was so surreal: You're on the water and snow is falling down and you're fishing in this beautiful area. It was fall and the leaves had turned color. I'm glad we went when it was cold and snowy. It was amazing, amazing."

"I got things out of the retreat I wasn't expecting. I got renewed. I feel so emotional about it: I had the time of my life, and the people were amazing. The whole atmosphere. And the beauty of the Salmon River, and the snow falling a little bit: It was perfect.

"I got new sisters. I feel like if I'm ever depressed or feeling bad I have someone I can call who really understands what I've been through, what I'm going through.

"I learned that our voices can be heard with the doctors. We're not like yes men: OK, OK, you're going to do this to me, you're going to do that to me. [Joanne Hessney] said, 'If you have questions or concerns, you can question your doctor.' A lot of women are scared and they don't do that. She gave me more authority with my treatment. I was having such severe side effects from the chemo, and Joanne taught me I don't have to suffer. Tell your doctor. Say, you know, this isn't working out for me. Can we try something else? She gave me the chutzpah to stand up for myself. Because you can get intimidated by your doctors. Every patient is different. Everyone's body reacts different."

Leslie, true to her upbeat nature, invested the stone she received at the retreat not with her fears and anxieties, but with sentiments of community and hope.

"It meant the togetherness we were all feeling, that we were all in this together. It was like a lucky charm. These are my sisters, and we're all in this together, and we're going to fight this thing."

Leslie hung on to the stone. She has it still.

Sue

"Going to Casting for Recovery, there was only one other woman there who was metastatic. When we were in a group talking about our cancer experience, one of the questions was, 'What's your greatest fear?' And we went around, and it was, 'Cancer coming back.' And I realized their greatest fear is being me."

Sue has short, curly, white-blond hair and twinkling eyes. She is fifty eight, appears vigorous, and is irrepressibly cheerful. The first thing you notice about her is her wide smile and easy laugh. The word that comes to mind to describe her temperament is "sunny." And yet.

"My greatest fear is dying. Their biggest fear is being me. I always thought we were on a continuum, and that's pretty true. But if the drugs stop working for me, the progression could be rapid."

She pauses for a moment. "It's all right," she says. "It is what it is. What are you going to do?"

She jokes easily about "cancer perks" and "playing the cancer card," and recalls how she learned about Casting for Recovery from a website with "cancer freebies."

"Dark humor suits me fine," she says. "I love to laugh more than anything."

When Sue was diagnosed, in the fall of 2014, she was, in her own words, riddled with cancer.

"I was metastatic when they found my cancer. So, I found out about it in this massive way.

"Thankfully, there are plenty of resources. I had a strong support network. Friends I could talk to. My husband's been great, my kids have been great." She and her husband have two daughters, one a recent college graduate, the other finishing high school.

Still, this was and is a diagnosis that could easily overwhelm even the strongest among us. *Everyone's* biggest fear is being Sue. We can only dimly imagine ourselves in this situation. It's a bit like wondering how we would react in an extreme emergency. Would we rise to the occasion, be courageous? Or would we go to pieces?

"I remember talking to my doctor before I was even diagnosed with cancer," Sue recalls. "My internist said, 'We're not going to have these results for a while. How are you doing?' I said, 'Fantastic!'

"You know, I have this really great ability to compartmentalize. And I don't think it's an unhealthy thing. I think it's a really healthy thing, because I'm not avoiding dealing with it. I deal with it. When it comes at me, I deal with it. But I can't be mired down in it, either. I can't live that way. I look at, I say, 'OK, I can't do anything about it right now. It's going over there.'"

Surgery, however, was not so easily placed "over there" and put out of mind. It was extensive and debilitating.

"I was flat on my back for eight weeks. The day-to-day was so overwhelming that I couldn't even think about the long term except to panic a little bit about the idea of more surgery or devastating chemo like you hear about."

Sue was at that time director of marketing for a large law firm, a demanding, high-profile job. She wanted to keep working, but she was living a new reality.

"I always thought of myself as pretty healthy. Diving, extreme walking, bungee jumping. I enjoyed that my body could do what I wanted. But, my cancer diagnosis…now I have some limitations. I went out on disability a little over a year ago. And I take much better care of myself now."

Sue has been recalibrating her life, helped along by her extensive network of friends and supportive family. She is, to borrow Sontag's language, negotiating her place somewhere on the frontier between the kingdom of the well and the kingdom of the sick.

"For the first year after my diagnosis, after I went back to work, I didn't want cancer to define me. The type of chemo I was on didn't take my hair; there were no external signs."

With a switch to a new medication, Sue did eventually lose her hair.

"It was really important for me to wear wigs and a hat. And I really resisted that outward display of my cancer, mostly because I didn't want that to be the first thing, like when you order a coffee and someone says, 'Oh, I'm so sorry about your cancer.' You just don't want that to be a part of every interaction.

"It was three or four months before Casting for Recovery that I just gave up with the scarves and the hats and the wigs. I was done with that."

Now, there was another step Sue needed to take.

"It took me two years to feel the need to go to a group, and Casting for Recovery did that for me. It was a kind of turning point where I realized that I should look for some connection within that community."

Sue attended the Casting for Recovery retreat on the Salmon River in 2016. She carpooled from Rochester with Sara. Like her, Sue was ambivalent about sharing her feelings with the other women.

"I wasn't excited about those parts of Casting for Recovery, but they turned out to be all right. My only anxiety about the weekend was sharing a room because I snore. I always bring ear plugs to share."

This takes a moment to sink in. Someone with metastatic cancer that could come roaring back at any moment and kill her is concerned that her snoring might keep someone awake? But this is in keeping with Sue's outlook about her disease, like her casual remark that, "It is what it is." She doesn't make too big a deal of it. When, during the opening night icebreaker at Casting for Recovery, she was asked to place herself in the stream mock-up and reflect on her emotional state for the other women, she picked a spot with "some action, but not crazy."

Sue especially enjoyed learning to cast on the lawn. Her instructor was Joanne Hessney, whose raucous sense of humor was to her liking. ("I'll pick the funny person first" in a group, she says.) Sue was a quick learner.

"On the river, we didn't get to do the full cast; we were doing side casting. And I thought, 'Hey, what's the point? I learned all this yesterday!' But it was so enjoyable to be on the river. It was such a beautiful, beautiful day. I'm so drawn to water. I could spend every minute on or near the water.

"I think the most wonderful thing about Casting for Recovery is trying something new. A very optimistic thing to do is to take up a new hobby.

"Fly fishing is something you can enjoy even if you're not really great at it. But the better you get at it, the more you learn. There's strategy and all the expertise you can develop. It gets richer and richer. Picking up something new that I'd never tried before and feeling good at it, it was a good feeling.

"I think it's a combination of the nature, the being immersed in nature because you really have to be someplace amazing to do it. The combination of the nature immersion and the competency, something you can develop competency in, and I've always enjoyed that. I can enjoy it at this level and then learn about the bugs!

"It was a wonderful experience: the fly fishing, the camaraderie, the openness. Better in the sense that it felt like a new chapter in reaching out, a new way to think about my cancer, a way to just keep growing in my coping with it. That felt like a turning point.

"Once you're faced with cancer, you deal with it a lot better than you think you will because you don't have much of a choice. If I've got six months, or six years, or sixty years, I don't want to piss it away by feeling sorry for myself and not doing things. I want to enjoy what I've got. I try to find ways to be happy."

Part 2.

Therapeutic Fly Fishing for Disabled Warriors

Chapter 7

Project Healing Waters Fly Fishing

Angling rehab for physical and invisible wounds

The victims of PTSD often feel morally tainted by their experiences, unable to recover confidence in their own goodness, trapped in a sort of spiritual solitary confinement, looking back at the rest of the world from beyond the barrier of what happened. They find themselves unable to communicate their condition to those who remained at home, resenting civilians for their blind innocence.
—David Brooks, "The Moral Injury"

Nearly a century ago, Ernest Hemingway published a short story that would help establish him as a leading literary voice of the "lost generation" of Americans coming home from the First World War. "Big Two-Hearted River" is about a veteran of that war apparently suffering from post-traumatic stress disorder, which at the time was called "shell shock." It is the story of someone struggling alone to recover emotionally from the horrors of combat that readers can only dimly imagine. But all of that is in the background and only hinted at. On its surface, "Big Two-Hearted River" is about a young man getting away from civilization for a few days of camping and fly fishing.

The story begins with Nick Adams, a Hemingway alter ego, arriving by train at Seney, Michigan, a small town recently destroyed by a forest

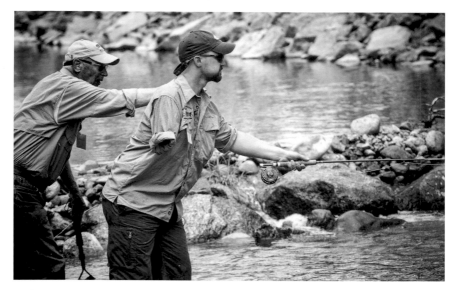

A disabled veteran learns to cast under the direction of a Project Healing Waters Fly Fishing volunteer. (Doug Buerlein, courtesy of Project Healing Waters Fly Fishing)

fire, which has left the landscape charred and barren: "There was no town, nothing but the rails and the burned-over country." A hotel has been obliterated. "The stone was chipped and split by the fire. It was all that was left of the town of Seney." The only place where life remains is in a river running beneath a bridge.

> The river was there. It swirled against the log spiles of the bridge. Nick looked down into the clear, brown water, colored from the pebbly bottom, and watched the trout keeping themselves steady in the current with wavering fins. As he watched them they changed their positions by quick angles, only to hold steady in the fast water again. Nick watched them a long time.

"Big Two-Hearted River" is considered the finest example of what Hemingway called his "Iceberg Theory" of writing. What we see of an iceberg is but a small part of its bulk, although we can imagine the roughly ninety percent of its mass below the ocean surface. Similarly, Hemingway's story focuses on surface details of a young man on a fly-fishing trip, while hinting at deeper meanings and motives, a submerged backstory. Not long into the narrative, we sense Nick has been through something devastating. Even the image of Nick hiking through the incinerated landscape suggests a lone soldier in a wasteland, holding his leather rod case like a rifle and bent beneath a huge pack on his back. He "took some of the pull off his shoulders by leaning his forehead against the wide band of the tumpline. Still, it was too heavy. It was much too heavy."

Nick leaves the town and turns "off around a hill with a high, fire-scarred hill on either side onto a road that went back into the country." He also seems to be leaving whatever is troubling him. As he hikes, "Nick felt happy. He felt he had left everything behind, the need for thinking, the need to write, other needs. It was all back of him."

When he arrives at the river, having passed through the fire-ravaged woods, it's as if he is returning to life.

> Nick looked down the river at the trout rising. They were rising to insects come from the swamp on the other side of the stream when the sun went down. The trout jumped out of water to take them… As far down the long stretch as he could see, the trout were rising, making circles all down the surface of the water, as though it were starting to rain.

"Big Two-Hearted River" has little in the way of plot: Nick hikes into the woods and camps overnight. In the morning, he prepares and eats breakfast, packs a lunch, gathers grasshoppers for bait, and fishes for trout. He focuses on individual tasks: finding a suitable campsite, leveling the ground, pitching a tent, putting up cheesecloth to keep out mosquitoes. The attention to detail seems to calm him, although there are hints that he is fighting demons.

> Nick was happy as he crawled inside the tent. He had not been unhappy all day. This was different though. Now things were done. There had been this to do. Now it was done. It had been a hard trip. He was very tired That was done. He had made his camp. He was settled. Nothing could touch him.

The following day, Nick fishes the river. He is a skilled fly fisherman, although, oddly for the twenty-first-century reader, he uses live grasshoppers as bait As in the first part of the story, Hemingway focuses on physical details as if he were a reporter. He describes Nick catching grasshoppers, stringing his rod, searching out likely spots for trout, wading into the current, casting, hooking, and landing fish. Nick is careful to wet his hand before touching a fish he plans to let go, "so he would not disturb the delicate mucus that covered him," a detail familiar to catch-and-release fly fishermen.

The quietly methodical way Nick goes about fishing for trout seems to bring him peace and a measure of control. Yet, there is a sense in the story that this control is hard-won, that emotions are roiling beneath Nick's self-confident exterior. After fighting and losing a big trout, Nick is shaken and suddenly unsteady: "The thrill had been too much. He felt, vaguely, a little sick, as though it would be better to sit down." For all his mastery of life in the outdoors, of camping and fishing, Nick seems almost fragile.

"Big Two-Hearted River" ends ambiguously. Nick seems more or less at peace, but an unspecific anxiety gnaws at him. He thinks about fishing in a swamp, but "Nick did not want to go in there now. He felt a reaction against deep wading with the water deepening up under his armpits, to hook big trout in places impossible to land them." The dark swamp where "the sun did not come through" seems to symbolize fearful memories the young veteran is not yet prepared to face As the story closes, Nick walks away from camp. "The river just showed through the trees. There were plenty of days coming when he could fish the swamp."

Hemingway chose fly fishing—Isaak Walton's "diverter of sadness,... calmer of unquiet thoughts"—near a post-apocalyptic wasteland as an emblem of the search for peace of mind by a veteran suffering from invisible wounds. In effect, Nick Adams undergoes what today is a bona fide "therapeutic recreation program for veterans with combat-related disabilities," that is, "therapeutic fly fishing (TFF)".[1] Among the benefits attributed to TFF are "reductions in PTSD (Post-Traumatic Stress Disorder) symptoms, depression symptoms, anxiety, negative mood states, and increases in leisure satisfaction and sleep quality."

For these and other reasons, fly fishing has become the centerpiece of therapeutic programs for disabled veterans and active military personnel. These include Rivers of Recovery, specializing in helping "combat veterans suffering with invisible wounds of war" by providing therapy and support during fly-fishing trips; and Project Healing Waters Fly Fishing, Inc. (PHWFF), which "is dedicated to the physical and emotional rehabilitation of disabled active military service personnel and disabled veterans through fly fishing and associated activities including education and outings," according to the organization's website.

PHWFF was started in 2005 at Walter Reed Army Medical Center by Ed Nicholson, a retired officer in the United States Navy and a Vietnam veteran. While a patient at Walter Reed, Nicholson came up with the idea of fly-fishing outings for recovering wounded and injured service members returning from Iraq and Afghanistan. The organization quickly took off. In 2020, PHWFF had 225 programs consisting of 9,765 disabled veteran participants and 4,295 volunteers.

PHWFF is a partnership between the U.S. Department of Veterans Affairs facilities and fly-fishing clubs, including Trout Unlimited, Federation of Fly Fishers, and independent groups. The program includes instruction in fly tying, rod building, and casting and offers guided fly-fishing trips. Everything, including tackle and other equipment, is free to participants.

Project Healing Waters, like all TFF organizations, relies on thousands of volunteers to plan, organize, and deliver its programs. One of these unpaid helpers is Kiki Galvin, a fly-fishing guide and personal trainer who lives in Virginia not far from Walter Reed National Military Medical Center, in Bethesda, Maryland. She became involved with PHWFF in 2007 after meeting Ed Nicholson at a fly-fishing show at the University of Maryland, and today is on the Board of Trustees. Galvin had been working with Casting for Recovery since 2000 and saw the transition to working with veterans with disabilities as a smooth one.

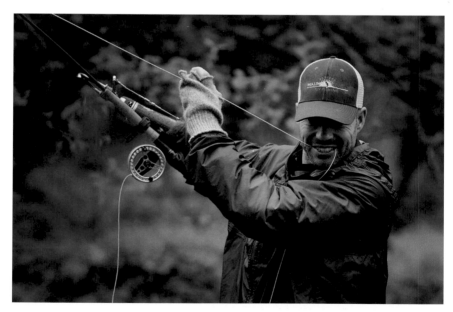

A veteran uses a modified arm prosthesis—and his teeth—to control the fly line. (Doug Buerlein, courtesy of Project Healing Waters Fly Fishing)

"There are parallels between these groups of individuals," Galvin says, comparing breast cancer survivors and wounded vets. "The women from Casting for Recovery have had trauma. They've had loss of body parts in some instances. They can suffer from PTSD. There can be a tremendous amount of depression. And our vets are pretty much trauma, PTSD, loss of body parts, and are on the same medications. In my opinion they are all warriors; they're just fighting different battles."

Galvin jumped at the chance to work with the veterans at Walter Reed: "It was very easy for me to say, 'Yes, I will reach out to a wounded vet or a vet who is in recovery' because I already understood the importance and the benefit I saw with people in Casting for Recovery. I knew how to reach out."

Every Wednesday Galvin drives to Walter Reed to meet with veterans during the noon hour at an occupational therapy center. Each session is devoted to some aspect of fly fishing—tying knots, entomology, tying flies, casting—depending on the time of year. Galvin also sometimes helps out on fishing retreats, although her guiding work can make the scheduling difficult. Regardless, she comes to know the vets and active military personnel over months and even years, as some are at Walter Reed for extended recoveries.

Galvin sees firsthand the physical benefits of fly fishing for those recovering from wounds.

"Fly fishing is very rhythmic and continuous," she says. "It's aerobic. It promotes circulation. It helps with rhythm and coordination. And when you are dealing with people who've had surgeries, with adhesions, injuries—a lot of just the physical casting promotes the healing process and promotes circulation. It also helps with balance and coordination."

But just as important is the camaraderie. Veterans who participate in Project Healing Waters, like the women who take part in Casting for Recovery, benefit from being with others who have had comparable experiences and are facing similar challenges.

"They are on a journey," says Galvin of both populations. "Once you've been diagnosed, once you're being treated, it's a new normal. It's a new journey in your life." TFF programs, she says, bring damaged people together in a "community of individuals who are going through the same things. Because sometimes they feel shut out from their family or their spouse, so you give them a population that is going through the same thing and it gives them a support group." This is especially critical in the recovery of wounded veterans, who speak often of their bonds with other warriors.

Many of the men and women who find their way into Project Healing Waters and similar programs suffer from PTSD, as Galvin points out. According to the American Psychiatric Association, people who have experienced or witnessed a traumatic event involving death, serious injury, or sexual violence may suffer from PTSD. Those with the disorder

> continue to have intense, disturbing thoughts and feelings related to their experience that last long after the traumatic event has ended. They may relive the event through flashbacks or nightmares; they may feel sadness, fear or anger; and they may feel detached or estranged from other people. People with PTSD may avoid situations or people that remind them of the traumatic event, and they may have strong negative reactions to something as ordinary as a loud noise or an accidental touch.

In just the past few years, a handful of researchers have turned their attention to the therapeutic effects of outdoor recreation generally, and fly fishing specifically, for those with PTSD.

PTSD has been treated with medications and a variety of therapies, including cognitive behavioral therapies, exposure therapy, and psychotherapy. Yet long-lasting positive results have been elusive for many sufferers.

Recently, however, alternative therapies, including outdoor recreation, have shown promise in helping those with PTSD. In one 2013 study published in *Military Medicine*, "Participation in Outdoor Recreation Program Predicts Improved Psychosocial Well-Being Among Veterans With Post-Traumatic Stress Disorder: A Pilot Study," researchers evaluated the effectiveness of two-day/three-night fly-fishing retreats for veterans with PTSD in alleviating their symptoms. The trips were run by *Rivers of Recovery*, which uses fly fishing "because the sport has been regarded to induce a calm alertness in a pristine natural environment that may enhance the ability to focus and reduce perceptual stress levels."

Researchers assessed participants' attentiveness, mood, depression, anxiety, and stress before, at the conclusion of, and six weeks after the retreats. They also measured PTSD symptoms and sleep quality at baseline and at the six-week follow up. "The primary hypothesis under investigation is that the fly-fishing retreat will predict acute elevations in attentiveness and sustained improvements in psychosocial well-being and sleep quality, in addition to reductions in PTSD symptomatology."

The *Rivers of Recovery* retreats include lessons in fly fishing and the opportunity for veterans to spend time outdoors with others fighting the same internal battles. The activity and environment are equally crucial to the therapy. Like Nick Adams in Hemingway's story, the troubled vets seek calm in an unspoiled natural environment and a sense of control in casting a fly line. The study authors include fly fishing among leisure coping strategies, which "have been argued to distract individuals from trauma." Also, "the calming environmental setting may serve as a grounding medium that enables participants to reclaim a sense of self unaffected by the combat experience."

This study was a pilot and included just seventy-four veterans, so its results must be read with those limitations in mind. Still, the authors' positive conclusions deserve to be quoted at length.

> The results suggest that outdoor recreation is linked to significant improvements in psychosocial well-being. Acute effects indicated significant elevations in attentiveness and positive mood states, accompanied by significant and sustained reductions in symptoms of depression, anxiety, and somatic stress, in addition to negative mood states. Moreover, the psycho-social benefits of the outdoor recreation appear to endure up to the 6-week follow-up assessment. Follow-up analyses revealed increases in sleep quality and significant reductions in perceptual stress and PTSD symptoms. An additional ancillary analysis revealed that reductions in PTSD symptoms served as a driving force that predicted improvements in sleep quality.

Or, in simpler terms, a weekend of fly fishing made veterans suffering from PTSD feel better and sleep better, and those benefits lasted.

Another study, published in *Therapeutic Recreation Journal* (2014), asked veterans to reflect, in focus groups, on their experiences during therapeutic fly-fishing retreats, which included fly tying in addition to fishing. The vets reported that the activities provided a way "to deal with the symptoms of their disabilities through distraction, focus, relaxation, and overcoming challenges and fears." They said they gained confidence and enjoyed a chance to feel normal. As with the veterans in the *Military Medicine* study, they benefited from the beautiful and peaceful outdoor environment. That being outdoors in a natural setting for a weekend "can foster both physical and mental well-being," as the study authors write, may seem an obvious conclusion does not detract from the apparent benefits to these men and women struggling with PTSD.

Broadly speaking, the therapeutic benefits of fly fishing in these pro-

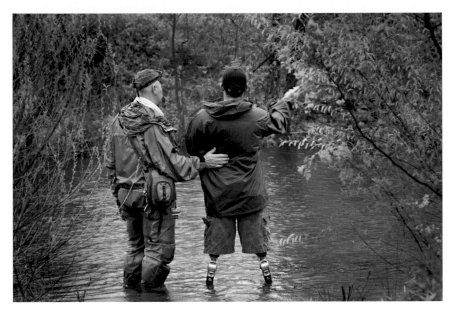

Project Healing Waters Fly Fishing is dedicated to helping veterans enjoy fly fishing regardless of physical disabilities. (Ed Feller, courtesy of Project Healing Waters Fly Fishing)

grams are twofold. First, veterans learn new skills, or adapt old ones to changed physical abilities, and practice them in a natural setting. As one observer writes of Project Healing Waters:

> The motions involved in fly tying, casting, and fishing provide physical therapy for torn and tattered bodies. Damaged hands respond nicely to fly tying; injured arms, shoulders, and backs get a wholesome and much-needed workout during casting, mending, and retrieving. Even more important, minds and hearts are refreshed by the tranquility of moving waters.

Second, and perhaps more important, participants find solace in the camaraderie with others facing similar challenges. "With the military, guys and gals in their battalion, it's like a brother- or sisterhood," Kiki Galvin says. "When they get injured and have to leave them to come back and be treated, they miss that camaraderie. So now you're gathering people in the military that have gone through the same thing. We're not replacing your battalion. But this is another group of individuals who have gone through the same thing [and who can] really support you."

People who take up fly fishing join a kind of fraternity, with its own language, lore, heroes, and secrets. That community has been especially welcoming of disabled veterans, offering a safe place to learn a new skill and enjoy fellowship in serene, restorative settings.

Notes

1. J.L. Bennett, M. Van Puymbroeck, J.A. Piatt and R.J. Rydell (2014). Veterans' perceptions of benefits and important program components of a therapeutic fly-fishing program. *Therapeutic Recreation Journal, 48 (2),* 169187. Retrieved from http://search.proquest.com.ezproxy.rit.edu/docview/1553177176?accountid=108, 171.
2. Bennett et al., 171.
3. In 2011, Walter Reed Army Medical Center was integrated with the National Naval Medical Center and renamed Walter Reed National Military Medical Center. It is located, as before, in Bethesda, Maryland.
4. E.J. Vella, PhD., B. Milligan, B.A., ans J.L. Bennett, M.S. (2013). Participation in outdoor recreation program predicts improved psychosocial well-being among veterans with post-traumatic stress disorder: A pilot study. *Military Medicine, 178*(3), 25460. Retrieved from http://search.proquest.com.ezproxy.rit.edu/docview/1348772224?accountid=108, 254.
5. In apparent agreement, the U.S. Government passed the Accelerating Veterans Recovery Outdoors Act, signed into law in December 2020, which establishes an interagency task force to promote the use of public lands and other outdoor spaces for veteran therapeutic activities and programs such as Project Healing Waters Fly Fishing.
6. Vella et al., 255.
7. Vella et al., 255.
8. Vella et al., 258.
9. Vella et al., 258.
10. Bennett et al., 175.
11. King, Montgmery. Fly Fishing, Fly Fisherman 39.4 (May 2008):3637, 5859.

Chapter 8

Maintaining Balance

Casting on the lawn at Fort Drum

This here, this isn't normal. —Kevin

It's noon on a warm summer day at Fort Drum, New York, and a dozen members of Project Healing Waters are gathered at Remington Pond. Every other Wednesday, when the weather cooperates, the volunteers meet there with vets and active military members to practice casting on the lawn and to fish the pond. On the alternate Wednesdays, the group meets at a sporting goods store to tie flies. Remington Pond and the small park surrounding it sit near the western edge of Fort Drum. Drum covers 168 square miles northeast of Watertown and is home to the storied 10th Mountain Division, which traces its history to troops on skis during World War II. The public relations folks there apparently have a sense of humor, calling "Drum Country," where winter temperatures plunge to -30 degrees Fahrenheit, "the warmest place you'll ever live."

Remington Pond is a peaceful green space inside a typical military installation, with mostly flat terrain, unobstructed views in all directions, roads running straight to the horizon, boxy living quarters, heavily guarded gates, and the occasional platoon of soldiers in fatigues marching in loose formation along a roadside. The men at the pond today talk about how much they enjoy this spot. They seem not to hear the occasional big gun going off in the distance. One jokes that once in a while they're buzzed by drones.

What the men stringing up their fly rods today have in common, in addition to combat experience, is treatment for Traumatic Brain Injury (TBI) and Post-Traumatic Stress Disorder (PTSD). They found out about Project Healing Waters while in treatment for TBI at Fort Drum. Today's group includes a father and son—the dad a Vietnam Veteran, the son nearing the end of his military career after multiple combat deployments in Afghanistan and Iraq; a soft-spoken young veteran, chunky and heavily tattooed, who is recovering from a gunshot wound to his face; a first-timer who just learned about the program; and a sixtyish veteran who looks so much like Ernest Hemingway that the others encourage him to enter the Hemingway look-alike contest held annually in Key West. Today someone brought a fly-fishing magazine for him with information about the competition.

Three of the men—the son, Kevin; the new guy, Bob; and the PHWFF organizer, Mike—stand together on the lawn, ostensibly to practice casting but mostly to kid around and listen to Kevin offer a jarringly lighthearted monologue about his military experience. He looks the part of the warrior he is. In his early forties, over six feet tall and about 200 solid pounds, Kevin has been a combat engineer for twenty years. His job is to ride around in an armored vehicle he describes as "a giant SUV on steroids" looking for Improvised Explosive Devices, or IEDs. Many have exploded beneath or next to his vehicle. He likes to say he's been blown apart and put back together again.

Right now, though, he's holding forth on hand-to-hand combat training. Recently he had to take a refresher course that he probably didn't need. He tells how a trainer picked him to demonstrate a technique.

"I know this stuff," Kevin says. "You get in close, keep in contact, never back up, never give up. I sort of kicked the guy's ass. The head trainer pulled me aside and said, 'OK, you're good. But you gotta let the trainers win.'"

The young man with the face wound has taken up a position on a pedestrian bridge over the pond and is fishing by himself. Others are laughing and telling their stories while occasionally sending a fly line across the lawn. Two men are seated at a picnic table comparing flies.

Kevin talks about how TBI has left him with poor balance. He can easily and unexpectedly become unsteady on his feet. Fly fishing has helped with this, so long as he is careful how he moves his head while casting, something he demonstrates as he works with a fly rod. If he were to keep his eyes on the line as it reaches out behind him, twisting his neck to watch, he could crash to the ground.

All this talk about equilibrium reminds one of the guys about a recent outing on a river when a wading vet's leg prosthesis kept floating out from under him in the current. "We went to work on it and figured out how to keep him planted there," he says, with a sort of unsentimental military can-do approach to a problem that's gotten in the way of a mission.

"Fly fishing also helps me with *balance*," Kevin says, gliding into metaphor. Angling and spending time outdoors with other injured warriors have brought him a measure of peace. He says the same of fly tying, which has become a passion for him as it has for many of the men and women who participate in these TFF programs. "It makes me focus," he says. "Everything else melts away."

Later, alone, Kevin opens up about his combat experience. He offers this history unemotionally and in minute detail. He has a habit of adding "and stuff" at the ends of sentences. This can make him sound like a high school kid recalling what he did over the weekend.

"I put in obstacles, clear mine fields and stuff," Kevin says. "We do breeching for urban operations. Since the War on Terror, especially when the IEDs came, we were the forefront of route clearing and finding the IEDs."

Kevin, a First Sergeant, was the tank commander of an armored "SUV on steroids," called a Buffalo, that his unit patrolled in while he was deployed to Iraq in 2006–2007. They were ambushed often. "Driven over multiple IEDs. Been hit by thirty-seven IEDs," he says, flatly, as if ticking off lines on his resume. "The very last one was the most significant."

Characterizing what happened as "significant" is like calling a heart attack inconvenient.

"It was at night. When you're doing route clearance, you're driving at about five miles per hour. You have twenty-plus floodlights on your vehicle, and there's like eight vehicles on that convoy, each with twenty lights on it. So, it's not like you're hiding from anybody." Kevin says this with a chuckle.

"We come up over a hill. So as we just crested over the hill and could see over, and there was an out-of-the-ordinary tree on the left side of the road that hadn't been there before. I was doing route clearance every day, from six hours to 18 hours, so you get to know the route."

Kevin was in the front passenger seat, next to the driver. A medic and mechanic were seated behind him. For everyone inside except Kevin, this was their first mission.

"I screamed out to stop, and he tried to stop. It's about a sixty-five-ton vehicle; even at five miles per hour it takes a good little while to stop. There was a copper wire across the road. It was a pressure switch, so it's, uh, victim operated.

"You're sitting up about 10 feet from the ground. When we had time to stop, we had rolled over it, and it blew up on us. It was a fifty-five-gallon barrel drum and basically a Claymore. They made it themselves. They had shrapnel in there. They had ball bearings about half an inch to an inch." He approximates the size by making a circle with thumb and fingers of one hand. A marble is a half inch in diameter. The IED exploded next to the driver's side.

"They had it angled up toward the windows. Shrapnel came through and went through my medic's arm. Big old shrapnel piece went through her arm in between the bone. Ripped the skin and everything from it. Went right through the armor. Another piece of shrapnel came in, hit the roof of the Buffalo, came down and went through my mechanic's thigh, through his calf, and pinned his foot to the floorboard of the vehicle. And then my driver, he ended up getting shrapnel in his shoulder. The ball bearings came through and went through his left ankle right at the ankle bone and destroyed his ankle bone. The whole ankle bone was gone."

Kevin can provide this level of detail because afterward he read a "blast analysis," a forensic reconstruction of the explosion and its aftermath. He cannot rely on his memory of the event. Some of that is lost because of what happened next.

"Two big old pieces of shrapnel came through, hit the windshield, came back, hit me in my, uh, basically like sunglasses, except with ballistic-rated lenses. I got shrapnel in the side of my head, in my nose, my lip, my shoulder. Another piece came through, hit the windshield, and came back and hit me right in the front of the helmet." The shrapnel broke the piece that holds night-vision goggles, shattered that, and lodged in his helmet.

"I was out for a good amount of time," Kevin says. "They were screaming my name 'cause they thought I was dead."

The blast "over pressure" sucked in his right inner ear. Kevin compares the feeling to the pressure in our ears when we fly, which we can relieve by working our jaw. He cannot make it pop. This is permanent.

"I came back to. I was in a daze. It was almost like a dream and you're trying to run away from something. But no matter how fast you run, you're really slow? It was like that the whole time.

"First thing I saw was my medic 'cause she was screaming, and she was right over me. And when I came to I saw her arm, and her arm was bleeding and all ripped up and stuff, so I put a tourniquet on her arm. I tightened it down just enough so that the bright red blood stopped."

Remarkably, given his condition and the chaos inside the Buffalo—"the person is screaming really loudly and stuff; they're in pain"—Kevin was following his training. Apply the tourniquet enough to halt the heavy bleeding, but not so much to cut off circulation altogether.

"I was able to save her arm from having to be amputated," says Kevin. He also patched up his mechanic, who kept his foot. Everyone survived.

How could he, as banged up as he was, manage to help the others?

"They're your brothers and sisters. You'll give your life for them. You're going to do everything you can to be sure they're safe and that they're taken care of."

Kevin is echoing what Kiki Galvin said about these warriors. They form bonds in combat that they miss when they return to the States or leave the military. "You'll never know brotherhood until you've had a brother lay down his life for you," Kevin says.

Now there is a hole in their lives. This explains why the men at Remington Pond spend so much time complaining bitterly about how the military bureaucracy has told them they have reached the limit on deployments. This makes no sense to Kevin.

"Here, you're not really contributing. You're not *there*. When you see the deaths on TV, you say, maybe I could make a difference. Maybe I could save lives. After a while that becomes normal. This here, this isn't normal." "Here" is a Dunkin' Donuts.

The men gathered at Remington Pond all are struggling with this new not-normal, which includes PTSD, Traumatic Brain Injury, life-altering wounds, damaged relationships, struggles with pain medication, dark thoughts. Listening to the chatter and laughter, it's easy to forget why the men are here, until the conversation drifts back to combat. This happens frequently. Anyone without their experiences might assume they would just as soon forget what they've been through. But they continually return to the same theme, the bond of brotherhood among warriors. They obviously miss the action and the battlefield solidarity.

The afternoon continues like this—working on casts, fishing a little (unsuccessfully), bullshitting, grousing about the breathtaking stupidity of the brass, enjoying each other's company. The men recreate for a few hours by a quiet pond the camaraderie so central to their well-being. They are pushing away demons, finding their balance.

Chapter 9

OASIS

Bob and Merilee Hoover are the sort of retired couple others aspire to be, living comfortably in their dream home on the shores of one of New York's Finger Lakes, Honeoye, with room for visiting children and grandchildren. They purchased the house, which needed a lot of work, on a whim almost 20 years ago when both were working as educators in local public schools. Married for more than fifty years, they talk in a sort of duet, not just finishing each other's sentences but switching back and forth to create sentences in tandem.

When Bob retired in 2006, he decided it was time to do something he had been thinking about for years. A former Navy Flight Officer who flew missions in Vietnam, he wanted to help returning veterans readjust to civilian life.

"We were getting the vets back from the wars and they were hurting," he says.

After research and long conversations with friends and family members, Bob and Merilee envisioned a program that would teach veterans with disabilities individual sports like skiing and fly fishing, get them outdoors, and continue supporting them as they rebuilt their lives. Their vision became OASIS, Outdoor Adventures for Sacrifice in Service[1], a nonprofit that assists veterans "in reconnecting and resuming productive lives in society through participation in outdoor recreational activities that promote independence, and social and emotional well-being." OASIS today teaches skiing, archery, sailing, rowing, golf, horsemanship, ice skating, and fly fishing, and serves vets from a six-county area in the Finger Lakes region. The service is free.

Getting OASIS to this point required prodigious amounts of energy and time, as well as a good chunk of the Hoovers' own money. The unavoidable question: What could motivate an enviably comfortable retired couple to extend themselves like that, to throw themselves into a project that for a while took over their lives?

"You have to go back to 1967," Bob says.

That year, Bob deployed to Vietnam as a Naval Flight Officer whose primary duties were as a bombardier/navigator. He left his new wife, Merilee, in California, where she attended college. While he flew missions over North Vietnam, she studied at California State College at Hayward (now California State University, East Bay). Their home was close to Berkeley, long a focus of political activism and, in 1967, the epicenter of the growing anti-war movement.

"We both experienced the bad effects of people in the United States not caring about what happened to people involved in the war effort," says Merilee.

She recalls, with irritation that lingers some five decades later, a California history course she was required to take in which the professor, in her recollection, spent less time on history than on criticizing the war.

"I quit going to the lectures," she says. "I was angry."

Merilee did manage to pass the final exam and the course. One day after the end of the semester, she ran into the professor on campus and he asked why she had stopped attending class.

"Because you started talking about Vietnam—my husband is there," she told him. "I have to believe that if anything happens to him that he's there for a reason. Obviously, you don't agree with that."

Although the professor "apologized all over the place," Merilee recalls, she had no illusions about changing anyone's mind. Neither did Bob when he returned from Vietnam in late 1967.

"I came back from that war hated," Bob says. "We saw what it was like to be hated. Back then, it was a different world. I was very careful not to talk about my experiences and my opinion."

"Because of the reception, that was something he always held in the back of his mind. That's not fair. That's just not appropriate," Merilee says.

These experiences planted the seed that grew into OASIS.

"He's had this in the back of his mind for a very, very, very long time," Merilee says.

Bob left the military in 1969 to attend graduate school, and he and Merilee went on to long careers in education. He was a middle school teacher, administrator, assistant superintendent, and education consultant; she taught physical education and health. Today, they still consider themselves educators, even in retirement, and OASIS has been an outlet for their drive to give others the tools to lead full, rewarding lives. In the beginning, when the idea began to take shape, all the Hoovers were on board. "The entire family was involved," says Merilee, "bouncing ideas off each other."

According to Bob, they asked themselves, "What do we want to accomplish? What do we want OASIS to do to help the recovery?"

The focus on sports came naturally, with Merilee's background in physical education and the couple's lifelong involvement with outdoor activities. They are avid skiers and fly fishers, among other things.

"We looked at sports, and I spent a ton of time on the computer researching," Bob says. "We were looking for sports that would allow individuals to see progress, but they would be trained with a team concept, surrounded by people," says Bob. "It's important for vets to understand they're not alone."

"We wanted to create independence in the vets," says Merilee. "We wanted to give them the skills and the support—whether it be in terms of equipment or transportation, whatever it was—so that if a vet woke up on Monday morning and said, 'I want to go skiing,' then he could do that."

Bob says, "The goal, I don't care what sport you're using, is to give them independence, confidence, and know they can get back into the mainstream of life."

The Hoovers searched for programs they could use as models but found nothing quite like what they had in mind. Their account of that process comes out in one of their duets: Merilee, Bob, Merilee, Bob.

"Looking at other programs for vets at the time, they're all these one-shot deals, and then, so long until next year."

"Basically, the vets say, 'This is great, but what do we do on Monday?'"

"We knew that our program had to be ongoing, not to abandon the vets and their families."

"We wanted it to be enduring."

They worked for two years, from 2008 to 2010, getting the program fully developed and filing the paperwork to make OASIS a nonprofit. The first class was in skiing at nearby Bristol Mountain Ski and Snowboard Resort, where Bob and Merilee had volunteered on the ski patrol for 26 years and were friends of the owner, Dan Fuller.

"We got the first sit-ski from Dan Fuller," says Bob. "Those things run five, six thousand dollars." That sort of generosity has propelled OASIS since the beginning. They've received donations and equipment from local businesses, as well as the use of sports facilities. A friend owns an archery range; that became the venue for classes in archery, the second sport OASIS added to its offerings. After five years, there were eight sports taught by 100 volunteers to 60 students, and Bob and Merilee could pass off the day-to-day management to the board of directors, although Bob keeps his hand in with the archery program.

The OASIS program has two phases. In the first, veterans learn and are guided in a new sport, typically over several months, including introductory classes. The objective is for the veteran to achieve independence in the sport. Cohorts are kept small, four or five veterans at a time, in part so each participant can be closely monitored.

Once veterans "graduate," they move on to the advocacy phase. OASIS works with the vet and with support organizations and individuals to help that veteran sustain independence in the new activity. In fact, the organization continually measures its own performance as well as that of the participants by collecting survey data from everyone involved. OASIS wants to see veterans achieve independence—a word that appears often in the organization's literature—in a sport as well as in their lives.

"We struggle bringing veterans into the program, and we struggle retaining them," says Tom Tartaglia, vice president of the OASIS board of directors and a former Marine. "When they're newly transitioning, they're going in a million different directions. 'Do I want to go to college full time? Do I want to work full time?'"

OASIS volunteers watch for clues that someone might be at risk to drop out. They also learn about PTSD, TBI, and sexual assault trauma so they can recognize and react to the anxiety and anger that can result from these conditions.

"Pull them aside," Tartaglia says, recalling instructions to the volunteers. "Don't single them out. Pull them aside and say, 'Hey, we're going to take a break. Why don't you come with us and grab a cup of coffee?'"

At the same time OASIS volunteers are watching for signs of upset, they are gently pressing the vets to be accountable. They have spent years, sometimes many years, in an environment where every second was accounted for, where they were ordered what to do, where to go, and when to go there. Readjusting to civilian life, where one's time is one's own, can be difficult for those who are more fond of their newfound freedom than they are of following schedules.

"We see a lot of accountability issues," says Tartaglia, who runs the archery program. "We give them parameters and we tell them, 'Hey, you're not going to be in the program if you don't show up on time.' They have to participate. They have a base level when they come into the program, and they have to show progress over time."

Regardless of these challenges, Tartaglia says most veterans stick with it because the rewards become evident to them quickly.

"One, they can learn to have fun again. During their time in the service, they might get into booze, possibly drugs. Sometimes it's the sheer excitement of jumping out of a plane. Or the exhilaration of a firefight. You get back to Rochester, and it's hard to find that sort of rush again. And that may be found in target shooting or skiing or fly fishing. We want these veterans to learn how to have fun again. Someone comes in and says, 'I'm afraid of the water,' and the next thing you know he's in the sailing program."

The second benefit, Tartaglia says, is community. "You get back home and you're going to school or in a job. It's not that brotherhood or that sisterhood that you had for that amount of time. We want them to learn appropriate transition tools so they can become a part of a community again that may not involve alcohol or may not involve drugs or some of the other habits they've learned." For the veterans, he says, OASIS is "like a tribe."

Fun, accountability, community, independence. These goals are a good match for fly fishing: having fun on the water catching trout; being accountable for your actions among other anglers (stream etiquette) and to the environment; enjoying membership in the community of fly fishers; and achieving independence in a sport that encourages and celebrates self-reliance.

When Bob and Merilee Hoover decided to add fly fishing to the course offerings, they sought out the help of two friends, Lindsay and Dave Agness. Lindsay is a well-known fly-fishing guide and instructor in the Rochester area. Dave, her husband and equally avid fly fisher, had been working with Project Healing Waters since 2005, so he had experience with veterans. In addition, both were involved with Casting for Recovery In 2013, the Hoovers asked the couple if they would run a fly-fishing course for OASIS, and they agreed to become program coordinators for what became known as "Fly Rod Warriors."

Each year, the Agnesses take on up to five vets for the class. They start in March with three indoor classes to teach the basics: tackle, appropriate dress, safety, stream etiquette, knots, fly tying, casting, and fly presentation. Dave and Lindsay work for Eastman Kodak; the company allows them to teach the class in one of its facilities. With classroom instruction behind them, and depending on the timing of the winter thaw, the class moves outside for fishing on at least four different area streams throughout the spring. Each veteran is matched with a guide.

"We have volunteers like Lisa Green who help throughout the

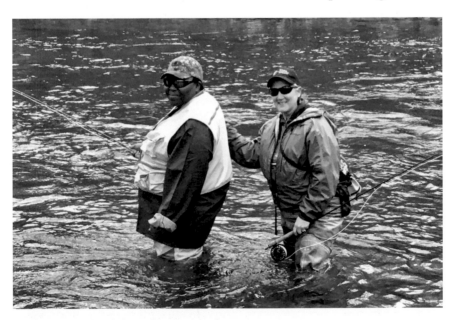

Lindsay Agness (right) on the water with a veteran.
(Courtesy of CompeerCORPS)

program," says Lindsay. "So if we have five vets, we have five guides on the water."

The Agnesses echo Tartaglia's comments about the challenges of participant retention.

Lindsay says, "The hardest part is getting them to show up for that first class. They don't know us, they don't trust us. We always lose one or two. We try to build up a rapport ahead of time. Sometimes you just can't get them out of the house."

The veterans come to the class, as they do to all OASIS programs, with some combination of PTSD, TBI, and physical disabilities, including missing limbs. Many are prone to bouts of anger.

"There's a lot of PTSD," Lindsay says. "They do check out once in a while; they have very short attention spans. They're looking at you and there's nothing there."

The participants are screened by OASIS, and the Agnesses have access to their medical profiles, as well as contact information for their doctors. This is a team effort, with each veteran connected to a network of medical and psycho-social professionals as well as volunteers. The support is critical.

Lindsay is convinced that, for the vets, taking up fly fishing and getting involved with the local fly-fishing community in a sense recreates their military family and sense of fellowship. The veterans, she says, "are used to having a very tight unit that watches their back. I think the fly-fishing community, as they go through this program, it's a very small group of individuals that are very close, and they all take care of each other. It's like a family, like that unit feel that they're used to. They can trust them."

Fly fishing, Lindsay continues, gives the veterans "a chance to bond and be part of a unit. What we're finding is, the ones who are feeling social and want to get out—not everybody's there yet—they'll go to Trout Unlimited meetings and be a part of that fly-fishing community, or they'll see them out on the stream, and they'll want to learn how to tie that next fly."

The Agnesses become very close to the men and women they instruct and guide. They make themselves available to them for casual fly-fishing outings and impromptu fly-tying sessions. "There are some vets where the fly-tying is more important even than the fishing," says Lindsay. As an example, Dave mentions a vet with PTSD who, when he becomes anxious at work, goes to a private area and ties flies to calm himself down.

"We have vets who never smile," says Lindsay. "But they'll get joy out of seeing someone else catch a fish. It's safe, it's the bonding, the sharing of their journey."

"We don't think about the challenges these guys and gals have to go through to transition back to normal life," Dave says. He speaks of one vet with "a lot of really intense anger issues" who told him, "I fight every day to figure out a reason not to kill myself. This program saved my life."

The veterans who join OASIS, like those who participate in Project Healing Waters, are damaged. Some have lost parts of their bodies; some have traumatic brain injuries; all of them suffer from PTSD. The country they have returned to is much more welcoming of vets than it was in 1967, when Bob Hoover came home from Vietnam. Yet they need much more than thanks and warm receptions. We can begin to understand the depth of that need by listening to the voices of these men and women as they reflect on their experiences and the support and comfort they have found in fly fishing.

Notes

1. At the end of 2020, OASIS merged with Compeer Rochester, Inc., and became a part of its veterans' services arm, CompeerCORPS.

Chapter 10

Voices of Veterans

*Veterans talk about combat, invisible wounds,
and the solace of fly fishing*

Over there, over there
Send the word, send the word over there
That the Yanks are coming
The Yanks are coming
The drums rum-tumming
Everywhere
So prepare, say a prayer
Send the word, send the word to beware
We'll be over, we're coming over
And we won't come back till it's over
Over there
—George M. Cohan, "Over There" (1917)

[Fly fishing] keeps me mentally occupied. I don't drift off to,
you know, over there.
—Dale (2017)

Over there, it didn't matter what you did.
You were never in control.
—Mark (2017)

Mark

In the months after 9/11, the three most revered professions were, in no particular order, firefighter, police officer, and soldier. Mark was all three then: a Rochester cop, a volunteer fire fighter in his hometown, and a medic in the National Guard. He has seen combat in Central America, Afghanistan, and Iraq. While he still fights fires, a few years ago, due to his severe PTSD, Mark was forced into retirement by the police department, and he left the military. But he still looks the part: tall and lean, with a military haircut. He is forty-eight years old.

Mark says that when he came home from his last deployment, in August 2013, "it" hit him.

"I became so isolated that my daughter would come home and say, 'Dad, you have to shower. You have to eat. Dad, you've gotta go do something.' It wasn't until then that I realized that I need help. That I need help bad. I went to the VA [Veterans Administration]. I went to the Vet center."

The VA judged Mark to be 70 percent disabled and essentially unemployable, although he has tried a few jobs. "But when my anxiety and depression hit, I don't want to leave the house. I call in sick more than I go to work. I've been trying all these programs. I tried a sleep study, I tried a parenting group, I tried all these different therapy groups, I tried meditation."

The answer, as for so many in Mark's situation, has been medication, a lot of it. He says the medicine is effective, "but I'm tired of taking six pills a day." He also has a service dog, a black Labrador Retriever trained by America's VetDogs®. "He senses my anxiety and depression," says Mark. "If I'm having a bad day, he will *not* leave my side. He will go into a dark room and turn on the light if I don't want to go in. He'll wake me up from a nightmare."

Today, sitting near the front door of a busy Starbucks, Mark is without his dog, whom he left at home because the weather is cold and the sidewalks are icy. People are continually entering and exiting, and the air is filled with the buzz of conversations, punctuated now and again with the barista's shouts and the clatter of plates. Mark says the setting is a bit of a challenge for him. By way of explanation, he recounts an experience in Iraq, in 2005, when he was attached to a counterintelligence unit.

"My whole team, we got trapped in a marketplace that was crowded. We were following a vehicle. We didn't ride in these nice up-armored Humvees. We were following a vehicle and turned a corner. And there's two of our vehicles, and the next thing you know we're in the middle of a marketplace."

Mark and the others in his car, fully armed, were dressed like local men and had beards and long hair. "If you stood me next to an Iraqi," says Mark, "you couldn't tell the difference between me and him."

The Americans found themselves trapped in the middle of a teeming, noisy, hostile crowd.

"Somebody spotted us, saw we had U.S. equipment. Shouted that we're U.S. And a firefight ensued. Just outside Baghdad. We were really lucky we got out. We were so jammed in there we couldn't get out the doors. We couldn't even get out the side windows. So crowds are not the best place to be." Not then, obviously, and not now.

Out of the military and the police force, Mark found himself with a lot of time on his hands, plenty of opportunities to brood, and few incentives to leave his house. ("Dad, you've gotta go *do* something!") This was when he learned about the OASIS program. An avid hunter all his life, he was attracted to the outdoor activities. He started with ice skating—he played hockey in high school—and then heard about fly fishing. He took the fly-fishing course with Lindsay and Dave Agness and learned how to cast and to tie a few flies.

"We went on a couple outings. And just like hunting, you're out there alone. It was nice just to be out there. I'm out there doing what I want, when I want. The other nice thing about it was I met a wide variety of vets. From Vietnam, Desert Storm, Iraq, Afghanistan. We had at least one common interest: the military. And now fly fishing is another common interest. And a big thing is listening to the stories about where to go, what fly to use, how to tie the fly.

"I was a woodshop geek in high school. So a big thing is building something and using it, and with fly tying I can do that. I can make my own flies and go out there and use them. It opened up a new chapter."

Mark enjoys the challenge of fly fishing, of mastering its complexities, and he especially relishes the security he feels when on a stream, either with friends or by himself.

"Safe and in control," he says of being on the water. "Over there, it didn't matter what you did. You were never in control. In Afghanistan, we had Afghans who had worked with us before. Went out on a mission, and because the Taliban paid them more than we did, [they] turned on us. So every sense of you being in control just went out the window. The entire time we were constantly wondering who's going to turn on us. We were constantly watching our backs. With the hunting and the fishing, we're in control. We feel safe because we're the only ones there. I don't have to worry about someone else. I don't have to worry about what's around the next corner."

Mark benefits from the camaraderie of fly fishing, but he usually prefers to be alone. This is not about fear of groups, though. Mark has always been self-reliant, although his independence has been undermined by the PTSD.

"The last couple years have been difficult because of medications. Between the highs and the lows, and the medication has been a huge trial and error the last two years. It's been an upward battle since I came back from my last tour. It's getting better day by day.

"I've been through two marriages because of all of this. But I have four wonderful kids."

All the children live with him, except for a seven-year-old boy from his second marriage, who goes back and forth between Mark and the mother. Mark also has a girlfriend now, although his struggle with PTSD gets in the way of that relationship. "If you asked my girlfriend, 75 percent of the time, I'd rather be without her than with her." This has nothing to do with who she is or what she means to Mark. He just needs to be by himself.

All this time in the Starbucks—while he talks about combat, his family, his adventures as a firefighter, and the mood swings that come daily—Mark is composed and a faint smile plays at the corners of his mouth. He becomes animated recounting how, in 2006, he successfully completed a live-hoist helicopter rescue of a family stranded during a catastrophic flood in Binghamton, plucking them from a deck as their house was about to float away. But when he begins to talk about his children, something changes.

"My son, all my kids, are a huge reason I haven't...." He pauses and looks at his hands, very briefly. "Why I haven't done certain things. They're the only reason I haven't done them."

He has regained his composure but continues to stare at his hands. The revelation that he has considered taking his own life is, in hindsight, hardly surprising given his history and the plight of veterans in the United States. According to the VA, veterans are one-and-a-half times likely to take their own lives as are non-veteran adults, when adjusting for age and sex. Every day in our country, about twenty vets die by suicide.

Mark is working hard to maintain his balance, to keep the dark thoughts at bay. He stays busy with the volunteer fire department, where he can enjoy the sort of comradeship and unity of purpose he knew in the military. And he gets outdoors whenever he can. Fly fishing has given him another means of reclaiming his self-reliance and finding peace.

"I have to get out," he says. "And it forces me to get out."

Mark is easygoing and pleasant to be with. He appears physically and emotionally sturdy, but clearly he is damaged, fragile. He is like a dam with deep, hidden flaws holding back roiling flood waters.

Dale

Dale is recounting the time he hooked into a steelhead. "BOOM! That fish was hot! That fish was *angry!*" He talks fast while he scrolls through photos on his smartphone, looking for pictures of the fish. He says "Dude!" a lot, either recalling a conversation with a buddy or for emphasis, as in "Dude, that fish was *angry!*" Words come out in bursts, sometimes in triplets, like when he quotes the guide's directions as Dale was fighting the fish: "'Come toward me! Come toward me! Come toward me!'" It's hard to know if this is a direct quote or just Dale's amped-up state. The volume is turned up just a little past normal, as well. He's wired like someone on ten cups of coffee.

Dale is thirty eight, married, the father of four young children, and suffering from "really severe" PTSD, the result of multiple combat tours in Iraq. He takes a lot of medication, which has made him gain weight. His hair is shaggy and he has a scruffy beard. He says he gets frustrated easily and is prone to bouts of anger. He cannot work.

"They don't want me working in the civilian world," he says. "I don't have the patience for ignorance."

Dale went to Iraq in 2003 and served with the 507th Maintenance Company. During the Battle of Nasiriyah, he was a driver in the same convoy with Jessica Lynch, who was captured and held prisoner until freed, famously, by American soldiers. Dale was a mechanic with a route clearance maintenance team, often riding in Buffalos in case of a breakdown. He did four tours in Iraq.

"When I got out of the military, I felt like I lost a part of my family, a part of me," Dale says. "I felt very alone. At times very short, very angry. I didn't have a purpose anymore. Everything slowed down." He also has flashbacks.

"A lot of times when I'm driving, I'll drift off and I'll think about what happened—relive some things over there. That used to happen a lot—to the point I was afraid to drive and would have my wife drive me everywhere. It triggers anger and guilt.

"My biggest problem is guilt. That's what my therapist and I are working on, trying to minimize that guilt. It already happened; you can't do anything about it."

When Dale came home from war, he got help at the VA Medical Center in Canandaigua, New York. He was assigned a social worker and, when she learned Dale is an outdoorsman, she sent him to OASIS. He tried his hand at archery and sailing, which he'd done as a boy growing up on Long Island. Then he told someone he'd like to try fly fishing.

"Dude said, 'I'll get you in. I'll get you in. I'll get you in.'"

Dale says he took to fly fishing instantly.

"I find peace," he says. "The sound of the water. Sometimes the cold air." But especially the thrill of hooking and fighting fish. Dale likes to say that "the tug is the drug."

He returns to his account of the angry steelhead, still shuffling through pictures on his phone. He was fishing that day with Dave Agness, who stood behind Dale, critiquing his roll cast technique.

"I was getting annoyed," says Dale. "I said, 'OK, drill sergeant.' I think Dave took that as his cue to lay off."

Dale is friendly and courteous. But there is something in his demeanor, something defensive, watchful. He seems aware of this. "You're on heightened alert" all the time, he says of his return to civilian life. This wariness, coupled with his restlessness, sends a message: Don't push too hard. Still, Dale is no loner. He especially enjoys fishing with other vets.

"I never fish alone. Because of my medical issues. In case something happens to me, I want someone to be there to call for help."

His favorite fly-fishing partner is a vet with two prosthetic legs. Dale carries a spare wading staff with him in case his buddy forgets his. His account conjures a vivid image of these two disabled veterans supporting one another in midstream.

"It gets me out," Dale says of fly fishing. "It keeps me mentally occupied. I don't drift off to, you know, over there."

It also keeps him connected. In fact, Dale has a link to the women of Casting for Recovery. He donated to the orginization, by way of Lindsay and Dave Agness, dozens of flies he tied. They attached one each to cards that Lindsay placed on the women's beds at the Tailwater Lodge to find on the first night of their retreat. The cards let the breast cancer survivors know that another kind of survivor was reaching out to them.

"I actually got a bunch of letters from them," Dale says, smiling.

Billie and Pam

They are a mismatch. Pam is big, overweight, and hobbled. She has a large knee brace on one leg and walks with difficulty. Billie is small and whippet thin and given to quick, bird-like movements. Pam talks slowly and deliberately, as though weighing each word. Billie speaks in excitable bursts but at low volume, each statement followed by a nervous laugh. Pam's voice is flat and unaccented; Billie's has the hint of a twang from her native Texas. They are inseparable.

"We're called Frick and Frack," Pam says.

The women, both in late middle age, met at the Vet Center for Readjustment Counseling in Rochester, where they were in therapy for PTSD. Pam had a job at the center, and Billie volunteered there.

"We were in the same program," Pam says. "We sat at the same table, we did our ceramics. We were side by side, and we didn't talk. It was like six or seven years before we spoke to each other."

This leads to a friendly argument as the two work out the chronology of their friendship. Billie says they didn't talk for six months; they go back and forth with corrections and recollections. They split the difference: three years in a program together without saying a word to one another.

"My years there were spent listening to every conversation," Pam says. "And there were a lot of guys there. So there were a lot of conversations I was listening to. Oh, we sat about as close as we are now focusing on what we were doing without…"

Pam's voice trails off, and she and Billie nod in silent agreement about their time in therapy.

"Don't trust people for a long time," Pam says.

They are seated at a small round table in a Starbucks next to a floor-to-ceiling window. Billie is in a corner; Pam has people behind her at a table.

"What's interesting is that when we're together, we basically have each other's back," Pam says. "Because right now she's in a safe spot and I'm not. But if somebody comes up behind me, I can tell by her face."

"Yeah, I keep an eye out," says Billie.

They are like soldiers on guard duty sitting on the ground with backs touching, watchful and mutually supportive, keeping each other alert. The conversation soon makes it clear each has gone through something harrowing in her past that remains present nonetheless.

Pam and Billie are reminders that while those with PTSD share symptoms—disturbing thoughts, nightmares, depression, anger, es- trangement—their trauma is uniquely their own. And the PTSD that veterans suffer from is not always combat-related and may have roots deep in the vet's past. They experienced or witnessed something acutely distressing: death, serious injury, or sexual violence.

The details of what these women lived through are clearly off limits. Yet each speaks vividly of her post-trauma experience.

"I started out with no memory of myself," Billie says. "I knew I had a family. I knew I had a daughter that I loved. I couldn't remember. That's where I started out. It took me a good 20 years to get to where I am now. It was slow going. I'd start these programs and then quit because it wasn't working. I'd get a great therapist and then she'd quit or she got transferred, and the trust went way down."

Billie punctuates these revelations with her nervous laugh.

"There was a time when I felt like sitting in a rocking chair and just dying," she says. "I spent five years in my house once, wouldn't come out at all. Just terrified. I used to think nothing affected me, but I guess everything did."

Frick and Frack have grown accustomed to speaking as a team. When one can't finish a thought, she looks to the other, and they work it out together. Here's how they describe their attitude toward life's bad breaks.

Pam: "You either make something good out of it or…" Billie: "…or you sit on your couch and die."

Both women have struggled with going out in public. After five years inside her home, Billie had to take baby steps to get off the couch, get to the door, go outside. Public transportation was an imposing hurdle.

Pam talks about forcing herself to get on a bus, with the plan that she would just ride it wherever it went.

"I got on the bus, walked down the aisle, got the hell off the bus!"

They break into a sort of call-and-response about their isolation.

"Grocery shopping at 2 a.m."

"Can't wait in lines. You start panicking."

"Usually takes me three years before I can talk to someone, before I decide to trust 'em. I'm better now."

"I'm working on it."

Several years ago, a counselor at the vet center referred Billie to OASIS. Billie mentioned it to Pam and soon they were enrolled. First Billie tried horseback riding and skiing.

"And I went to fly fishing, and I went, 'Found it!' I like wading in the water. I like catching the fish. I like tying the flies."

"The flies we make look like nothing on this planet," Pam says.

The women don't think much of their casting skills, either. But none of this seems to matter. They've found in fly fishing a reason to be outdoors and among people, and a means of escape from the mental prison of PTSD.

Billie says, "It de-pressurizes me. Sometimes I'm not even fly fishing. I'm sitting on the bank enjoying nature. It calms my mind. My mind runs in a hundred different directions at once. And I go fly fishing and I'm instantly calmed down, and I focus on what I have to do to catch that fish.

"It just energizes me. The freedom. When you hook one, it's all the excitement. Pitting yourself against that fish. And just the quietness of the woods, and the people. I'm usually a loner, like her. But I'm getting better, a lot better. It just kinda brings me out of myself. I want to be around these people. I don't understand it fully."

"Yeah," Pam says, nodding in agreement, although she's more inclined to be on her own. "You're out there casting and it calms you down, and you don't care if you catch a fish or not. I love getting out in the middle of a river, a lake, whatever. No people around. Just quiet. I love that. Get me out in nature. The sound of the animals. And when you're there by yourself, that's it. It's safe. It's calming. It's you and maybe just a squirrel or a chipmunk, and they don't sass back."

Billie and Pam took the OASIS fly-fishing class with Lindsay and Dave Agness and have become close to them. But at first, the instruction was difficult because of the physical contact. Pam recalls a session on fly tying, which typically involves a standing instructor leaning over the seated student from behind to show how it's done.

"They'll come up behind you and say, 'Now, put the thread back.' And I'm like: You are behind me. I don't do well with behind."

"You gotta see 'em," Billie says. "And you don't even know this person."

"The first time you come up to someone you don't trust him," says Pam.

"It took a long, long time for me to let people get this close to me," Billie says, thinking back to those classes. "It took me a while because they have to get close to you. I got used to it after a while when I knew they weren't going to kill me or maim me or something."

She laughs again. A listener is tempted to think she's joking or at least exaggerating. But this is coming from a woman who for five years could not leave her house, who is afraid of waiting in line, who wanted to die.

If their fly-fishing experience has helped Pam and Billie relearn how to trust, they credit the many volunteers.

"The volunteers that do this, they're wonderful. They're just wonderful," Billie says.

Pam jumps in with, "Yeah!"

"I don't know where they come from, but they're like angels," Billie says.

"Yeah! And they're so patient. And they take their time. And what I love is, every time they say something, it's always positive. There's no negativity."

Billie says, "Sometimes I'm looking at them and thinking, 'Are you for real?' My experience with people is they're just pretending. They're going to go around the corner and start laughing at me. You know, the PTSD...."

Part 3

Therapeutic Fly Fishing for Those Recovering from Addiction

Chapter 11

Moving Meditation

How fly fishing complements treatment for addiction

Be happy in the moment, that's enough. Each moment is all we need, not more.
—Mother Teresa

Many men go fishing all of their lives without knowing that it is not fish they are after.
—Henry David Thoreau

"It is about focused attention. By focusing your attention on, say, what your fly is doing, the rhythmic motion back and forth of casting a fly line, it creates a sense of centeredness and calmness, very similar to what happens in meditation."

This is Steve Hanna, a licensed professional counselor and clinical addiction specialist, reflecting during a phone interview on how fly fishing helps people in their recovery from addiction, substance abuse, and depression. Hanna is a fly-fishing instructor and guide for Four Circles Recovery Center, in the Blue Ridge Mountains of North Carolina, an "adventure-based addiction treatment center offering drug rehab programs & substance abuse recovery for young adults," ages 18 to 28. Four Circles promises its clients a "transformational journey of self-discovery" by way of challenging wilderness activities, such as canoeing, rock climbing, whitewater rafting, and fly fishing, in combination with 12-step-based therapies. In tune with the healing philosophy of Four Circles, Hanna embraces the transformative power of nature, especially when it includes handling a fly rod. He views fly fishing as a sort of vigorous meditation.

"There's active meditation and there's passive meditation," he says. Think of the latter as someone sitting on the floor in the Lotus position, eyes closed. "This is more an active meditation. You're paying attention to what your body is doing and what it feels like to have your arm moving through the air, and that focuses your attention: on walking in the river, on paying attention to the hatch."

Like others who link fly fishing with meditation as a source of stress reduction and centeredness, Hanna is a proponent of mindfulness. Mindfulness is being completely aware of one's thoughts, emotions, or experiences in the present moment, and accepting each without judgment, moment by moment. It involves learning to accept unpleasant feelings like cravings, to explore those feelings in the present, and to let them pass.

The authors of a 2016 comprehensive review of studies of Complementary and Alternative Medicine (CAM) for addiction write that "Meditation, mindfulness or yoga have been suggested as being effective for the treatment of addictions; and there might be several plausible mechanisms of action involved. For instance, studies have shown that mindfulness meditation limits experiential avoidance by interrupting the tendency to respond using maladaptive behaviours (i.e., substance use)." Or, in simpler terms, mindfulness meditation could be helpful in recovery from addiction by relieving stress and helping addicts resist cravings.

Addiction to drugs or alcohol is a chronic disease that is notoriously resistant to treatment. The National Institute on Drug Abuse puts the relapse rate for drug addiction at between 40 and 60 percent. Even worse, according to the National Institute on Alcohol Abuse and

Alcoholism, approximately 90 percent of recovering alcoholics will relapse at least once within four years after treatment. These discouraging statistics, along with the high costs of addiction to individuals, families, and society, have led to myriad treatments that complement conventional medical and psychological therapies. These CAM options include acupuncture and its variations—auricular acupuncture, auricular electro-acupuncture, auricular laser-acupuncture, acupressure, electro-acupuncture—herbal medicine, hypnotherapy, mindfulness meditation, music therapy, spirituality, traditional Chinese medicine, yoga, and more. CAM use by patients struggling with addiction is high, ranging from 34 to 45 percent.

It is safe to say the jury is still out on the effectiveness of CAM in treating addiction. The review of studies cited earlier suggests the evidence is "contradictory" and "confusing; or negative." Yet, mindfulness meditation stands out as central to many addiction treatment options, so much so that practitioners often refer to Mindfulness-Based Stress Reduction (MBSR) and Mindfulness-Based Relapse Prevention (MBRP).

According to a recent study of complementary therapies for addiction, "Mindfulness trainings, which are based on ancient Buddhist psychological models, have recently been tested as addiction treatments and have yielded promising results. Fascinatingly, these Buddhist models revolve around the elimination of suffering, which is thought to be the inevitable product of craving." "The primary goal of MBRP," write the authors of another study of mindfulness and addiction, "is to help patients tolerate uncomfortable states, like craving, and to experience difficult emotions, like anger or fear, without automatically reacting."

"Mindfulness is about changing your relationship to your emotions," says Hanna. "And seeing that your emotions are signals about things that are going on, and that they're temporary. And if we just stay present, they kind of pass on their own."

Fly fishing is Hanna's way of staying present, of focusing on the moment-by-moment immersion in technique and moving water. "What it's like to have your feet cold and the rest of your body warm," he says. "It's kind of a body-centered awareness." That is, moving meditation.

Angling with a fly rod in this case brings the same or similar healing benefits and sense of well-being seen with cancer survivors and disabled warriors. These include exercise in calm-inducing surroundings, focus that offers troubled minds a respite from anxiety, self-assurance that comes with mastering a difficult task, and a sense of camaraderie and common purpose among people in similar circumstances. In addition, fly fishing is a ready source of apt metaphors.

Four Circles Recovery Center promotes angling as "rich with metaphors for life in recovery," offering therapists "opportunities to explore the issues underlying each client's substance abuse." Hanna is adept at mining fly fishing for such metaphors and making them a part of stream-side counseling of young men and women struggling with addiction.

"When you dry fly fish, there's the drag that happens, so you're mending your line so that you're presenting the fly naturally," he says, providing an illustration. "The same thing happens in moving meditation: When my mind wanders, I mend my mind, I bring it back to the present moment." At this point, Hanna begins to imitate his presentation to clients as they fish. "So this is how we're casting, how we're breathing, how we're being careful wading through the water."

Programs like Casting for Recovery and Project Healing Waters Fly Fishing also draw on metaphors from fishing to illuminate the inner lives of people recovering from physical and emotional wounds. But those figurative linkages are not as central to healing as they are to Hanna and others working in his field. For them, metaphors are the very basis of therapeutic fly fishing. Hanna practically riffs on the metaphorical opportunities, beginning with the most elementary of fly-fishing skills.

"Knots are about connections," he says. "They remind us about our connections with ourselves, with other beings. And with a higher power, or something bigger than us. And when they're tied properly, they maintain our connections even when stress is put on them. If they're tied improperly, or we put too much pressure on them, they break or sever, and we lose our connection."

Picture Hanna speaking these words as he teaches a small group of clients, standing and sitting by a burbling creek amid the Blue Ridge Mountains, how to tie a fly to tippet with an improved clinch knot. This is therapeutic fly fishing at its most evolved, where everything—river, fish, line, knots, cast—becomes a mirror that reflects the inner life, a metaphor of some facet of recovery. Hanna takes the knot metaphor to another level:

"So when they're tying a blood knot, I get them to think about their relationships with their immediate family, their blood relatives. And how has their addiction broken those ties, how does their recovery bring back that connection?"

Hanna's use of fly-fishing metaphors is reminiscent of the meaning-making of Rabbi Eisenkramer and Pastor Attas in *Fly-Fishing—The Sacred Art: Casting a Fly as a Spiritual Practice*. Eisenkramer connects the trout stream with a ritual bath in the waters of life, *mayim chaim*. Attas, a cardiologist, links the river with life-sustaining blood. If Hanna's metaphors are less overtly religious, they are similarly spiritual. He seems to use the metaphors to draw out his listeners, to help them see their experiences in a broader context, to move beyond the personal to the universal.

Hanna is clearly excited by the possibilities of these connections and of passing along the habit of metaphor-making to his young charges.

He recalls a rainy-day fishing outing at Four Circles during which he came upon a young man sitting by a stream apparently doing nothing.

"He was watching the water droplets disappear into the river. It reminded him of how he had taken water for granted, and he had to filter water for 30 minutes just to get a cup. He got an appreciation of natural resources being limited. So he was getting some bigger sort of self-in-universe perspectives."

This anecdote of a fly-fishing epiphany brings to mind Reina, the Casting for Recovery participant who virtually lived inside a metaphor during her first fly-fishing experience. The moving water was for her a reminder of chemotherapy, but that image was transformed into something cleansing, renewing.

For Steve Hanna, fly fishing continually offers up moments like this that can be epiphanies for the angler and therapeutic material for the addiction counselor. Part of his role is to help clients be mindful of those experiences as they happen.

"I'm going to give you a quote," he says. "When I heard it, it just struck my heart. What this gentleman said was, 'Fly fishing isn't about going to the river and making things happen. It's about discovering what's going on and becoming a part of it.'"

Notes

1. P. Posadzki, M.M. Khalil, A.M. Albedah, O. Zhabenko and J. Car (2016). Complementary and alternative medicine for addiction: an overview of systematic reviews. *Focus on Alternative and Complementary Therapies, 21*(2), 69-81. doi:10.1111/fct.12255, 78
2. Posadzki, et al., 70.
3. Posadzki, et al., 78, 79.
4. S. Houlihan and A. Judson (2016). The emerging science of mindfulness as a treatment for addiction. In E. Shonin, W. V. Gordon and M. Griffiths (Ed.), *Mindfulness and Buddhist-derived approaches in mental health and addiction* (191-210). Switzerland: Springer International Publishing, 191.
5. S. Khanna and J.M. Greeson (2013). A narrative review of yoga and mindfulness as complementary therapies for addiction. *Complementary Therapies in Medicine, 21*(3), 244-252. doi:10.1016/j.ctim.2013.01.008, 247.
6. The blood knot, also called a barrel knot, is used to connect lengths of leader or tippet. Before the advent of tapered leaders, multiple blood knots were used to tie together leader segments of gradually decreasing diameters. Some have suggested that the resulting multi-segmented leader's resemblance to a cat-o-nine-tails gave the knot its sanguine name.

Chapter 12

Rainbow's End Recovery Center

Once in a while you just have to get away. Away from schedules and responsibilities and whatever is eating at you, away from the beeping and jangling, the relentless hustle of work, to somewhere far removed from the familiar, somewhere *different*, where the pace of living slows from a sprint to an amble, where you not only can relax but get reacquainted with yourself.

If you feel the need for that sort of escape, you could do a lot worse than to get yourself to Custer County, Idaho. Named for a mine which

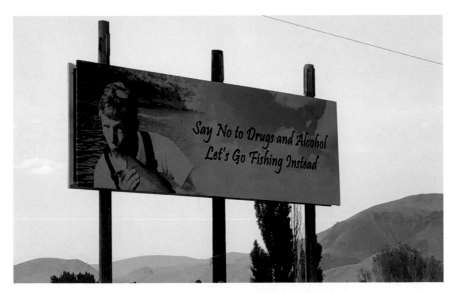

A billboard near Rainbow's End Recovery Center, in Challis, Idaho, promotes fly fishing and sobriety. (Photo by Patrick M. Scanlon)

was named for the luckless general, this territory near the center of the state is about the size of Connecticut and home to just 4,300 people. That's a population density of 0.9 Idahoans per square mile (Connecticut's density is 739; Manhattan's, 70,826). With a straight face, Wikipedia refers to Challis (population 1,000) as the "largest city" in Custer County, of which it is the seat. More reasonably, the local Chamber of Commerce calls Challis a "small town with a big heart," and a Wilderness Gateway. A short drive from town, usually on one of the rugged four-wheelers that are parked everywhere, is the Salmon-Challis National Forest and "some of the most pristine wilderness in the continental United States."

Challis sits almost exactly one mile above sea level. This is high desert. There are sagebrush and cactus, as well as mule deer, elk, and bighorn sheep that stand and stare down from narrow ledges on the barren hills around town. Drive or walk out of Challis a short way, and you are alone in a vast landscape with a view for miles in every direction.

This is a place to get lost—figuratively, if you need to; and actually, if you're not careful. Place names say it all. The Lost River Range, with peaks of 11,000 and 12,000 feet, runs southeast from near Challis for 75 miles. To the east of the mountains is the Little Lost River; to the west, the Big Lost River. More or less bisecting the state and flowing past Challis is the Salmon River, which has long been known as the River of No Return. It gets its name from a particularly unforgiving 200-mile stretch between the outposts of Salmon and Riggins, where its swift current tumbles between canyon walls that slice through roadless back country. As early explorers, including Lewis and Clark, quickly learned, you can boat in but not out the way you came. You either take to land or just keep drifting through the 2.36 million-acre Frank Church-River of No Return Wilderness, the largest and among the most remote and rugged wilderness areas in the Lower 48.

The Salmon River is less treacherous and considerably more accessible where it meanders and braids its wide way north past Challis, with U.S. 93 running alongside it and matching its bends. Take that highway out of town, and after seven miles of seeing not much, you'll spot a lone billboard on the right. It displays a photo close-up of a young man in waders standing in the River of No Return, holding and kissing a large rainbow trout. Bold cursive text that seems to appear out of the sky in the picture reads, "Say No to Drugs and Alcohol. Let's Go Fishing Instead." Just beyond that sign on the right, a driveway passes between two stone pillars that support a delicate wrought-iron arch with the words "Rainbow's End" curving rainbow-like overhead.

Rainbow's End Recovery Center comprises a cluster of houses and outbuildings on a verdant lawn that runs down a short hill to the river. Behind the main house is a paddock for the resident quarter horse, Cocoa. Next to a meeting house—the capacious interior furnished with overstuffed chairs and exercise equipment, and dozens of humongous replicas of fish adorning the walls—is a small pond with a fountain at its center. The water is filled with chunky rainbow trout that boil the surface like piranha when food pellets are thrown at them, as happens throughout the day. The compound resembles an upscale, private summer camp or a bed and breakfast, which at one time it was.

Rainbow's End is a residential drug and alcohol treatment facility offering extensive one-on-one attention to a small number of clients matched by a nearly equal number of counselors. The official capacity is around a dozen, but since the center opened in 2011, there have never been more than seven or eight residents at one time. Clients share rooms for two, with separate lodgings for men and women.

"You are here to be treated for your drug and alcohol addictions, not punished for them," reads the center's website. The therapeutic approach at Rainbow's End is laid back, personal, non-judgmental, and holistic. The goal is to help clients live their lives in a way to avoid drugs or alcohol dependence, and treatment includes guidance in self-discipline, budgeting, paying bills, and eating well. Treatment draws on the "12 Steps" but also on "peaceful restorative activities in a serene environment." These include hiking, rock hunting (Idaho is the Gem State), and fly fishing, either in the backyard pond (where success is a certainty) or the Salmon River, which is just a few steps away. As the Center's promotional literature states, "Piscatorial therapy"—less ostentatiously, fly fishing—"has proven to be a highly effective treatment for anxiety disorders."

Nancy Del Colletti is the executive director of Rainbow's End, although she likes to call herself "a combination of an administrator and your great aunt." A retired public-school teacher from California, Del Colletti opened the center with her husband, Aly Bruner, who introduces himself as the guy who cuts the lawn. They originally bought the place to open a bed and breakfast but later decided on a change when a counselor friend told them the spot was perfect for a recovery center because of its calming, restorative setting.

"It's been pointed out to me by energy healers that this is a very special place," says Del Colletti. "I'll accept their beliefs—it works for me. There's a vortex of energy that comes from the mountains that's kind of pointed in this direction. And people that are real empaths can feel it."

It's hard to know how seriously to take these comments. Del Colletti has a disarming way of conveying, alternately, hard-headed pragmatism (the administrator) and New Age mysticism, always with genuine warmth (the great aunt) and flashes of good-natured irony. As she might say: Whatever it takes to get the message across. This is consistent with the Center's approach to treatment. The counselors help people in recovery by using whatever works: poetry, music, meditation, long walks, grooming Cocoa, watching the golden eagle that nests on the opposite shore of the river—anything that calms the client and draws him or her away from brooding on the past or worrying about the future.

For addicts and alcoholics desperate (or forced) to get sober, getting away—from the surroundings, routines, people, and temptations that feed their addictions—often is essential to their joining the community of the recovering. They need a peaceful spot a long way from home, a quiet, uncomplicated, healing place far from the using crowd.

On this day in early August 2017, there are seven clients in residence at Rainbow's End: four twenty-somethings—two men and two women; a woman in her early thirties; and two women in late middle age. A few of the current residents know the center well: This is their second visit. Two in the group are preparing to leave in the coming week; two arrived just a few days ago and look edgy and disoriented.

"You watch people come here from cities, and they are so wound up they don't know how to go a day without electronics," says Del Colletti. "We take their phone away for the first seven days. They are just beside themselves. They can't function. But then once they realize that they can go outside and walk around, they can throw a fishing line, they can throw rocks in the river, they can do other things with their time, and it opens their eyes a little bit and relaxes their mind. There's a peace to coming anywhere there's nature."

Not long after Nancy and Aly opened Rainbow's End, as they thought about how best to take advantage of the setting, they learned about an organization that used therapeutic fly fishing to treat veterans with PTSD, and they immediately saw the possibilities.

"These organizations seemed to be cropping up everywhere," Del Colletti says. "It's that whole Walden Pond thing where you just go out and absorb the whole atmosphere around you and realign your rhythm to the rhythms of nature. It's not just the rhythm of the casting but the rhythm of your breathing. If you align your breathing to your casting and that slows you down, it takes the edge off."

Rainbow's End highlights therapeutic fly fishing in its promotional literature and on its website as central to the Center's experience. The

Salmon River is the "perfect atmosphere for healing and recovery from drug and alcohol addiction." Fly fishing "requires timing, patience and discipline, all skills which help in a person's recovery from drug and alcohol addiction." It is a "contemplative activity" and "comparable to meditation.... When standing in the river, one concentrates on nature, fly fishing and playing the fish. Your mind shifts into a lower gear; the rhythm of the river and casting help reduce anxiety and tension."

But angling doesn't work for everyone, and no one at Rainbow's End is pushed to pick up a fly rod.

"A lot of people will choose meditation on a rock as a form of mindfulness," says Del Colletti. "But fishing is natural to this area and very calming. I've tried it myself."

Among the counselors is Jed, who is sixty-two and drives between his home in Challis and Rainbow's End on an impressive Harley-Davidson. Short, bald, and bearded, Jed is deeply tanned but turns crimson when he's excited or laughing, which is often. He speaks slowly and sparingly—a common response to questions meant to draw him out is "Yep"—and many of his sentences are rounded off with a chuckle. He was heavily into drugs before getting clean twenty-five years ago.

"I came to work at this facility because they have fly fishing as therapy," says Jed. "For me, this was a great way to combine my work with my passion."

Jed is a fly-fishing guru. For him, angling is not only therapeutic for those in recovery; it's a healing respite from a world that's moving too fast for us to keep up.

"It teaches people how to live in the now. Keep their head out of the past. Keep their head out of the future. Helps them to be present in the moment right now, to connect with the world around them. Brings them back and grounds people... in the moment. And that's huge. Most people struggle with staying in the moment. In our society everything is so fast-paced anymore. Everything is go, go, go. Pick up a fly rod and all that disappears. And just live in the moment: the water, the fish, the air.

"There's nothing I like better than to sit on the river all day fishing. I could stand on the river starting in the morning and then suddenly it's dark, and I wonder where the day's gone. And I'm calm and totally at peace. It's my reconnection with the world."

Jed is sitting on a patio near the trout pond. He frequently gestures at the surroundings, at the river bending out of view and past dusky hills that rise from either shore, at the trees along the opposite bank. Once he breaks off in mid-sentence to point out an eagle flying into a tree nearby.

"Life around here is very peaceful," he says. "You might call it slow because you're so used to all the stimulation from the traffic and the people and the movement. And you come out here and it's gone. And your senses are in shock because it's very quiet here. The quiet here is almost loud."

Jed is no fan of the city.

"The busy-ness: We're not designed to live like that. I think we're designed to live in peace and harmony with the planet."

For many of the clients who are struggling to adjust to sobriety, finding harmony and calm can be a challenge. This is especially the case for those who are not yet committed to changing their lives, a not uncommon condition, according to Jed. Some residents have trouble just sitting still. For Jed and others at Rainbow's End, the moving meditation of fly fishing offers a path to mindfulness that is itself a pleasurable physical outlet and stress reliever, a way to discharge dark psychic energy.

He says, "We talk a lot about mindfulness around here. We teach them how to breathe, get that nice breathing going. Then we teach them to cast and get a rhythm with the breathing and the casting. And they forget about the past and stop worrying about the future.

"When you're totally in the moment and you're fly fishing, your mind is on the motion of the fly rod and the rhythm of the cast. Emotions just disappear, and you become one with what's around you. Like I said, you're not in the past, you're not in the future, you're not living off an emotion unless it's the excitement of fishing. It's about letting go. This is how simple it is to let go. You get mindful and into the moment. Packing these problems around does not solve them. Staying upset and worried does not fix anything. To let it go is key to everything."

Everyone at Rainbow's End—counselors, clients, the office assistant, even the barrel-shaped house dog that rarely moves—seems to live in the moment. There is a schedule of activities neatly laid out in a spreadsheet on the Center's website, with every minute of every day accounted for. But a visitor quickly learns that the timetable is more aspirational than dictatorial, except for the meals and morning and afternoon group sessions that anchor each day. Clients are kept busy, yes. But flexibility is the watchword. Whatever works.

"I try to live in the moment all the time," says Mitchell, fifty-seven, another counselor. "Someone once asked me, 'How do you plan out your day?' 'Well,' I said, 'lunch is at noon.' I go with the vibration of the day. You know where I am right now? Right now I'm right here with you. I'm talking to you. I'm not anyplace else."

Mitchell, also a recovering addict, is stocky and has close-cropped hair and a wide grin. He is perpetually serene.

"My supervisor once told a client, 'Mitchell is the only person I know who is constantly in meditation,'" he says.

His attitude makes Mitchell a perfect fit for the accommodating treatment philosophy at Rainbow's End.

He says, "Spontaneity is what it's all about. I'm not rigid. I go with the flow. Everything I do with people has to have flow in it. If it doesn't, it's not real. If there's not flow involved in what we're doing, it becomes false. It becomes a lie. It becomes part of our rigid societal view of how things are supposed to be. 'I'm supposed to be this, and I'm supposed to be that.' I try to open their eyes up to the possibilities of flow. That it isn't this and that. This and that are lies. Illusions. Reality is *this*."

OK. This takes some getting used to, especially for anyone who keeps a calendar. And Mitchell can come across as, well, a little off the grid. But going with the flow at Rainbow's End *is* what it's all about. That and mindfulness, and time on the river.

"When you bring somebody into the present moment, that's what it's all about," Mitchell says. "Fly fishing is a present-moment thing. They're fly fishing. They're not thinking about the past, and they're not thinking about the future. They're right there in the moment. You bring them into the present moment of fly fishing, and you tell them, 'Look at what you're doing right now.'"

Mitchell describes, as did Jed, teaching clients to cast and breathe in sync, to get into a calming, centering rhythm.

"But it ain't all about that," says Mitchell. "I teach them a whole lot

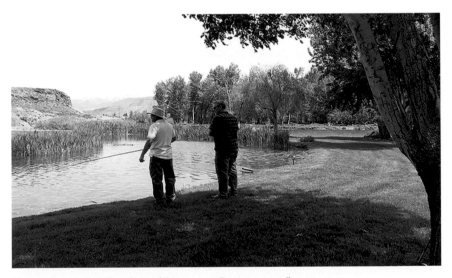

Counselors at Rainbow's End Recovery Center enjoy "moving meditation" while fishing the center's trout pond. (Courtesy of Rainbow's End Recovery Center)

of ways of finding their center. Programming yourself to understand meditation. All different kinds of meditation. We don't always have the opportunity to fish because the seasons get in the way. But when we have the opportunity to fly fish, we do it. We're not always in charge of it. Sometimes it's them on their own doing it. The pond is there; it's full of fish."

Clients choose Rainbow's End for different reasons, among them the remoteness and quiet, but many come here specifically for the fly fishing, some from as far away as the East Coast. Experienced anglers are already well on their way to achieving mindfulness, according to Mitchell.

"If they are fly fishermen, they already understand it without even knowing it. And then I introduce them to different kinds of breathing exercises. Different kinds of visualization. If they're fly fishermen, they already understand what it is to be mindful. Mindfulness—what it means to be present in the moment—can be difficult. But if they already understand what it is to fish, they're already there."

"Fly fishing," Mitchell says, summing up, "is a way to take us away from the suffering of life into a peaceful place."

As Jed said, they talk a lot about mindfulness around here: about being present in the moment, forgetting about the past, not worrying about the future. For counselors at Rainbow's End, as for Steven Hanna in his work on the other coast, the moving meditation of fly fishing is a sort of portal to a state of emotional equilibrium and calm, a means of achieving what Hanna calls "a body-centered awareness." Besides, it's an excellent stress reliever.

In the afternoon, some of the counselors and Del Colletti are chatting in a reception area of the main house, where there are overstuffed chairs and a desk. The room is situated between the kitchen and one of two front entrances, and as the staff talk and check their smartphones, clients pass through on their way into Challis for an Alcoholics Anonymous meeting, accompanied by another counselor. Mitchell has been describing some of the ways he tries to engage clients.

"What we're trying to find is what works for each individual," he says. He mentions taking clients out rock hunting. "I haven't done it so much since I stepped on a rattlesnake."

One of the residents leaving for the meeting, a young woman who has recently returned for a second stay after a relapse, stops before Mitchell with her arms outstretched, and he rises to give her a bear hug. There's some friendly joking about her having all the materials from the previous visit, which was only a few months ago. The staff are happy to see her, in a bittersweet way. This is a relapse, after all. In a moment, after a quick catch-up, she and the others are out the door and off on the short drive to Challis in the Center's van.

It is profoundly unfair that all the harmed people in this book face shame. The veterans and active military personnel struggling with post-traumatic stress often feel they have let their comrades down. If they are away from the action, they are not doing their duty. (Kevin: "This here, this isn't normal.") They may see themselves as malingerers, a perception reinforced by cruelly oblivious and uninformed others who view PTSD as a sign of weakness. Cancer survivors are isolated and singled out by the disease. The emblems of their sickness and its treatment, particularly the lost hair, are there for everyone to see, and too frequently the reaction is to avoid eye contact or the obvious topic of conversation. In this way, the cancer survivor can become an outcast, a walking symbol of our own fears, a damaged human being linked with a metaphor for malevolence. (Sontag: "The people who have the real disease are... hardly helped by hearing their disease's name constantly being dropped as the epitome of evil.")

Shame is particularly acute for addicts and alcoholics. Although attitudes are slowly changing, as research continues to demonstrate how substance abuse is an illness, too often addiction is seen as a moral failure and a sign of weakness. It's what people with flawed characters do to themselves. They aren't attacked by a cruel, indiscriminate disease or traumatized by heroic combat. They brought this on themselves. Add to the impact of such misconceptions the grim reality of relapse rates, which, as we saw earlier, range between 40–60 percent for drug addicts and 90 percent for alcoholics within four years. When everyone knows you're in recovery, falling out of it is an especially public humiliation.

Recovering addicts and alcoholics live on the razor's edge every day. The precariousness and embarrassment of their situation often is the subject of their conversations, of the stories they tell about struggling to get better.

Chapter 13

Voices of Recovery

*Addicts reflect on the restorative
powers of nature and fly fishing*

Josh

Josh, forty-eight, stayed at Rainbow's End for the first time in late 2016. He was sober for six months after that. Then a romantic relationship went south and he relapsed, quit his job, sold his house, and made his way back to Challis for a second visit. It was, as he recalls during a phone conversation, "the epitome of starting over."

A lifelong angler, Josh was delighted with the Center's location on the Salmon River, but fly fishing was secondary to his choosing Rainbow's End.

"It certainly didn't hurt," he says. But what attracted him primarily was the laid back, summer camp vibe. "I would've been a caged animal elsewhere."

Still, Josh fished whenever there was an opportunity.

"We'd have group outside, and when we had free time afterward, I'd fish."

Sometimes Mitchell and Josh would go to a lake nearby for some fishing and counseling.

"I've always enjoyed fly fishing, I'm passionate about it. But until I sat down with Mitchell, I never really understood the meditative properties or how relaxing it is.

"Prior to Rainbow's End I wasn't the kind of person who practiced Eastern philosophy, meditation, Buddhism, Taoism. Mitchell introduced me to some of those. As I kind of got into meditation, it would bring my heart rate down, my blood pressure was lower. When he pointed out in his office that you can meditate while you're fly fishing, a light bulb kind of went on in my head. It's more than the sound of the river and getting into that nuance and rhythm of casting, it's like— yeah!—it... kind of put a completely different perspective on it for me so that the next time I picked up my rod after having that conversation with Mitchell, I had a newfound freedom and different perspective on the whole concept of fly fishing that opened up why I really liked it."

For Josh, fly fishing had been a means to get away from what was troubling or pressuring him. In that respect, it had something in common with alcohol.

"I used fly fishing prior to Rainbow's End as a kind of escape. I was out of cell phone range, I wasn't distracted by personal relations, I wasn't distracted by work. But I was using. So it kind of shined a light for me that I truly love fly fishing, but now I love fly fishing sober. Because before, I was using it as a crutch to get away and to isolate, which I did in my addiction, whether it was fly fishing or locking myself in my house with a couple bottles of wine. It was just another form of isolation. Now for me it's truly a form of rejuvenation.

"There's a centeredness about fly fishing. Whether I go fly fishing alone or with someone, I'm alone because there's a distance between me and my partner. It forces you to think without distraction. It forces you to explore your internal 'me.'

"I'm about three minutes from the Boise River, and I've spent a few evenings casting until dark. For me it's just that consciousness that, yeah, I want to catch fish, but now I want to get more out of fly fishing. There's that meditation and relaxation, and the centeredness and focused breathing."

He doesn't use the term, but Josh is practicing Moving Meditation. The experience leaves him relaxed and renewed.

"You know how you feel after you get a physical massage? After I've packed up my vehicle, I feel like I got an emotional massage. And because of the emotional relaxedness, your body feels great. It's a Zen-like state."

Josh talks about how other clients at Rainbow's End were fascinated with fly fishing, even if they didn't take it up. They would watch him casting on the river or pond. He recalls one of the women saying, "'Wow, I could just sit here watching you cast! It's beautiful.'"

In this way, fly fishing became a springboard for therapeutic give-and-take. Without being aware of it, certainly, Josh acted as a sort of stand-in for Isaac Walton, holding up angling as "a calmer of unquiet thoughts, a moderator of passions, a procurer of contentedness." His transparent love of angling prompted clients watching him cast to reflect on their own means of finding peace and calm.

"They said they could see why I love it so much, and they started inquiring about what I get out of it. It was dialogue, not monologue, and they were interjecting what relaxes them. It was a conversation."

That conversation continued after he left Rainbow's End recently to begin his dream job, booking worldwide fly-fishing adventures for an outfit based in Idaho. He talks on the phone to one of the current residents, Amy, nearly every day.

Amy

"I would sit and watch Josh fly fish, and the art of it. To me it's beautiful. I just always think I can't do it. But I thought I couldn't do a lot of things coming here."

Amy is rail thin. She sits with her legs crossed, a femur starkly visible through the fabric of her shorts. After thirteen years of sobriety, recently she relapsed and eventually landed in a hospital intensive care unit—weighing 80 pounds. ("I don't eat when I drink.") She was malnourished and covered with bruises from a damaged liver. Today, relaxing in the sun near the trout pond at Rainbow's End, Amy has a worn and brittle appearance; her face is drawn and faintly lined. Especially seen from a distance, she could be taken for either a teenager or a woman in her fifties. She is thirty-four years old.

Amy entered what she calls an "addict-help-addict confrontational" recovery program when she was twenty-one and already a late-stage alcoholic. There was a lot of shouting and humiliation. She lived there for two years and then stayed on as an employee for another eleven.

"Working there daily with clients, I lost, you know, myself."

Then the bottom fell out.

"Why the hell, after being sober for thirteen years, did I stop at a gas station and pick up a drink one day? I'd been divorced, my mother had died."

Amy returned to her family ranch in central Idaho to help her dad, who was left adrift after the death of his wife. She also returned to drinking, always alone.

"I'd reach under my bed in the morning, drink to stop the shakes. I had very severe 'DTs' (Delirium tremens, an alcohol withdrawal symptom characterized by shaking, confusion, and hallucinations). And I knew my dad was going to find out. So in a drunken fear I tried to commit suicide. I would rather die than let someone know. I would rather have died than face the shame and guilt. I thought that would be my wake-up call. Two days later, I was drinking again.

"That whole concept of emotional sobriety, I didn't have that that entire time."

So, she made her way to Rainbow's End.

"I came here and it looked like a resort. I could sit outside all day now. Before, I couldn't stop fidgeting.

"So much of emotional sobriety is spiritual, emotional well-being. Learning here about the different aspects of spirituality: It's nature, it's around you, it's the aura, it's the sounds, it's the breathing."

Today is Wednesday. Amy checks out on Saturday to go back to her father's ranch, 3,000 acres on the Big Wood River, where they grow alfalfa and barley. It won't be easy living in a small, tight-knit community or attending AA meetings in a place "where everyone knows your junk."

"This isn't my first rodeo, so I feel prepared for what I'm about to face. I feel like I've formed some good habits here."

"The constant practice of what we've learned here of listening, of being in touch with your spirituality, learning about the different types of Buddhism, of Native American types—we burn sage to cleanse—those little things. I have this new confidence."

Seeking perspective on her own "junk" is what drew her to sit by the water at Rainbow's End and watch Josh casting a fly line.

"I can see the therapy in the breathing and the strokes and the art of it. And being one with the water and the fish. I see the grace of it. To me, it's the breathing. I've been so high-strung out of my addiction that a deep breath is the greatest thing for me. It feels so good."

Ethan and Noah

Ethan and Noah are recent arrivals at Rainbow's End, although this is Noah's second stay this year. They sit across from one another at a picnic table outside the meeting house, both looking shell shocked. Ethan is twenty-three and was partying pretty much non-stop as a college student until he was arrested. That led to community service, drug and alcohol classes, and thirty days at Rainbow's End. Noah, twenty-five, dropped out of school "to become an addict instead." He was forced by a court to come to Rainbow's End the first time, about six months ago. This time was his choice.

Conversation is difficult for both of these young men; words come haltingly. Noah struggles to make himself clear. He frequently apologizes for his inability to express himself.

Noah: "My family is all fly fishermen at heart, and white water rapids. In my addiction, I don't want to be fly fishing unless I'm loaded. Now I want to do what the normal thing is and maybe I'll enjoy it. Oh, man, it's a drug in itself. Just the stillness."

Ethan: "I grew up fishing a lot. I got away from it. I think something good about it—not just me, I think most people—trying to involve their drugs or alcohol with all their activities. You know, if I'm going golfing, I'm drinking. Like, whatever you do, everything involves your drug or alcohol. So here, fly fishing is something you can do that takes you outside while being sober."

As Ethan is talking, the two young women clients walk by in swimsuits, headed down to the river for a dip. Without a word, Noah gets up to follow them. Ethan stays a while to chat but never seems at all comfortable. When the women pass by again wrapped in towels, with Noah in their wake, Ethan excuses himself and joins the group.

All four seem even younger than they are, as if drug and alcohol abuse had somehow suspended them in their teens. And they appear utterly lost, especially the guys, so recently arrived and trying to find their bearings. Youth, with all its promises of future fun, may be working against them.

Bob

"I'll tell you the therapeutic aspects and the not-so-therapeutic ones. "The therapeutic aspects of fly fishing are that it is an absolutely wonderful sport into which you can lose yourself completely, and it takes the place of addiction in so many different ways. You don't miss the ritual of drinking. It occupies your time, your mind. It stimulates the pleasure side of your brain. It's by its very nature therapeutic. Being outdoors and noticing the world around you is something addicts don't do very much. They're usually confined to a space and their own little world.

"The downside is the social aspect of it. If you go fly fishing here in the Catskills, you don't stop when it gets dark. You stop at a bar, which is what probably 60 percent of fishermen do. That is the downside. The socializing after fly fishing becomes an important part of the ritual of drinking."

Bob, who lives on the East Coast, is calling from the Catskills, where he's been fishing, with little success, the Willowemoc Creek and Beaverkill River. In his seventies, Bob has enjoyed a distinguished academic career in the sciences, with hundreds of publications to his credit and several university administrative positions in his past.

"And I did that with a bottle of scotch on the table. I was perfectly happy being an alcoholic. Drinking was a complex part of a ritual."

His complacency with drinking was not shared by his family, who intervened to guide him toward recovery. They discovered Rainbow's End and assumed it would be a perfect fit for Bob, a lifelong angler. He spent thirty days there in 2016.

"There was actually a lot less fly fishing than I thought there would be because there's so much time spent on serious aspects of therapy.

"Fly fishing is a very important part of my life. I realize now that I can do that, and I am doing it in such a way that I'm enjoying all the positive aspects of it that are helping me avoid the negative ones. I don't feel any desire to connect with other fishermen at a bar."

Bob has an intriguing history with alcohol and fly fishing. He has never mixed them.

"I never, ever drank while fly fishing. That was like an unspoken rule for me. And I never fly fish alone. I have a very good friend, and we would spend a couple weeks every year going various places fly fishing. We never drank. We would pack in for a couple weeks and we would be completely dry. We looked at it as a chance to detox."

"When I was at Rainbow's End, the therapeutic sessions helped me see how I was (a) in denial and (b) reinforcing all my bad habits by perpetuating rituals I didn't really have to do to enjoy myself. It was beneficial for me to quit. Rainbow's End really helped me see the aspects of what I was doing that inevitably affected my ability to really understand myself.

"The people there—even the cook—they all are just extremely helpful in terms of getting you to see the aspects of yourself that are preventing you from enjoying the rest of life free from drinking. I realized for the first time in my life that drinking was hurting me and I really wanted to stop."

Mitchell and Jed introduced Bob to mindfulness and breathing in rhythm with his cast.

"That's their specialty. It's vaguely Jungian. We had lessons that we read and you had to participate in discussing them. A lot of them are Jungian in terms of symbolism, in terms of self-awareness, mindfulness. We discussed synchronicity.

"Mitchell is the more philosophical, although Jed is, too. They both really stress getting to know yourself, getting to know the positive aspects of yourself, starting to really think about yourself, and stop to think about the world around you.

"First you have to love yourself. You have to realize you have to do something positive for yourself. You can't do it alone; that's why you're in therapy. You have to realize those parts of yourself that are preventing you from understanding yourself. Don't worry about the past, and don't worry about the future. There's absolutely nothing you can do about the past, and absolutely nothing you can do about the future. Jed used to say, 'If you have one foot in the past and one foot in the future, you're pissing on today.'"

Bob took quickly to the notion that fly fishing is a means of blocking out past and future, of being alive to the present.

"When you're fly fishing, you have to concentrate on taking the next step and not slipping on a rock. You have to position yourself to be able to cast to a rising fish. You have to get to a spot where you can reach that fish without scaring it away. Everything is... what are you going to do with your very next move. There's nothing else where you're so much in the moment, except maybe a boxing match. You can't think about what happened yesterday, that's for sure.

"It wasn't just me fly fishing. Jed would take us out—you can't just take a bunch of addicts out who've never fly fished and have a positive experience; it just won't work. But we could have a therapy session outside by the pond, and Jed would show the rudiments of setting up the rod and how to cast. And he would have me show people the motions. Almost all of them were interested in the concept of fly fishing, and it's a whole lot better than being in jail or hounded by someone. Having those therapy sessions outside was a very pleasant experience. It worked very well for being in the moment... connecting with yourself and feeling positive about yourself."

A year after his time at Rainbow's End, Bob is still sober.

"The thing is, you can't really fish for trout if you're buzzed."

Part 4

How Fly Fishing is Therapeutic

Chapter 14

The Green World

How being in nature heals us

Thousands of tired, nerve-shaken, overcivilized people are beginning
to find out that going to the mountains is going home.
—John Muir

Contact and connection. That is what my passion and need and
obsession for mountain rivers, for wild water and wild trout is all
about—the deep ache to be joined again, even if for a passing moment, to the natural world, that part of life in which everything is
whole and united, mountains and rivers, trout and human beings.
—Harry Middleton, *The Bright Country: A Fisherman's Return to
Trout, Wild Water, and Himself*

Trout don't live in ugly places.
—Anonymous

In 1863, Frederick Law Olmsted traveled from the East Coast to
California to manage the Mariposa Estate and gold mine north of
San Francisco. The following year, the United States Congress passed
the Yosemite Grant, which required the state of California to hold a
large territory, including the Yosemite Valley, in the public trust "for all
time." President Abraham Lincoln signed the grant into law. Due to his
reputation as co-designer of Central Park in New York City, along with

some helpful political connections, Olmsted was appointed chairman of a commission charged with overseeing the new park.

Imagine Olmsted's first encounters with the soaring peaks and spectacular vistas of Yosemite after years living and working in New York City and Washington, D.C. Before coming west, he had served as executive secretary of the U.S. Sanitation Commission, a forerunner of the American Red Cross, which was responsible for the well-being of Union soldiers. The father of American landscape architecture had been transported from an increasingly urbanized East during the darkest hours of the Civil War to a timeless wilderness of ethereal beauty.

Olmsted, who also was a successful journalist, vividly described the park in a report, "The Yosemite Valley and the Mariposa Big Tree Grove" (1865). He proclaimed Yosemite the "union of the deepest sublimity with the deepest beauty of nature."

> No photograph or series of photographs, no paintings ever prepare a visitor so that he is not taken by surprise, for could the scenes be faithfully represented the visitor is affected not only by that upon which his eye is at any moment fixed, but by all that with which on every side it is associated, and of which it is seen only as an inherent part. For the same reason no description, no measurements, no comparisons are of much value.

Olmsted knew the park would be a tourist attraction, in fact wished to encourage visitors, but he was concerned that over time, human traffic would despoil it. He proposed roads, trails, and bridges, along with structures for hikers and campers, which would provide access with as little alteration to the landscape as possible.

Olmsted's fellow commissioners weren't impressed. They buried the report, and the designer headed back east to resume a brilliant career. But "The Yosemite Valley and the Mariposa Big Tree Grove" remains a testament to a vision that was central to the development of our system of national parks. Natural scenes are not only breathtakingly beautiful, but also, and more importantly, restorative and reinvigorating to over-worked and anxious Americans, who at the time Olmsted's report was published, were emerging from a horrific war. Olmsted argued that going into nature is fundamental to an inalienable right, the pursuit of happiness.

> It is a scientific fact that the occasional contemplation of natural scenes of an impressive character, particularly if this contemplation occurs in connection with relief from ordinary cares, change of air and change of habits, is favorable to the health and vigor of men and especially to the health and vigor of their intellect beyond any other conditions which can be offered them, that it not only gives pleasure for the time being but increases the subsequent capacity for happiness and the means of securing happiness.

Anyone who reads all the way through Olmsted's report quickly realizes there really aren't many "scientific facts" in it. He writes, for example, that the pressures of business (for men) and household cares (for women) can cause "softening of the brain, paralysis, palsy, monomania, or insanity." Somewhat mystically, getting outdoors would help set matters right.

Most likely, Olmsted relied for his conclusions on anecdotal evidence, tradition, and his own experiences. But here's the thing: He was on to something. A mountain of recent and ongoing (truly) scientific research has established a strong link between being in or near natural environments and good physical and mental health. Nature really *is* good for you.

The notion that the natural world has a nearly magical ability to return us to mental and physical health is an ancient one, explored in art, philosophy, and religion for centuries and across many cultures. This connection was particularly strong during the Romantic movement of the early nineteenth century—when Frederick Law Olmsted came of age—as artists and writers, reacting to the Industrial Revolution and the growth of cities, celebrated nature, as in the poetry of Wordsworth and Shelley, Longfellow and Whitman. Ralph Waldo Emerson made "Nature" the title of his founding essay of Transcendentalism (1836); and his neighbor, Henry David Thoreau, sent millions of late-twentieth-century Americans into the woods with *Walden* (1854) tucked into their backpacks.

Returning to ourselves by going away to a simpler natural world, fleeing the busy-ness and complications of our social entanglements and responsibilities, is a kind of cultural touchstone. It is a common theme of Shakespeare's comedies—think of *A Midsummer Night's Dream*—in which characters escape an oppressive society and head into a forest, a supernatural "green world" where problems are resolved, truths revealed. The changed individuals, usually young men and women previously at odds and now united in love, return to an altered society where the natural ordered has been restored.

Today, we, too, go to green spaces, whether a mountain forest or a city park, to remove ourselves for a while from the stresses of modern life and to recoup our energy and emotional equilibrium. Being in nature is not just an escape; it is an opportunity to unravel complications, to reset our lives, and to start over refreshed.

The belief that time away in a green world calms and comforts stressed human beings has been confirmed by a growing body of research grounded in evolutionary psychology. Because our species evolved for most of its history outdoors in nature, modern human beings "are not fully adapted to urban environments and… something may be missing when we are deprived of contact with nature." We spend more than 90 percent of our lives indoors or traveling from one building to another, according to the U.S. Environmental Protection Agency, yet we retain an abiding connection with the natural world.

More to the point, we respond to natural settings in a way that is, in a word, healing. We come away from the green world—shifting here from poetry to scientific prose—"with an increase in our positive affect and decrease in our negative feelings or stress—particularly when we have interacted with those environments that were favorable for our survival as a species."

What are those favorable environments? Contact with almost any green space has therapeutic benefits. It "can lower stress levels, restore powers of concentration, and alleviate irritability," according to one study. However, research has shown that we are least stressed when in a place that in our long history as a species would offer safety, particularly where there are visible horizons and a body of water. One prominent study of our aesthetic preferences in natural settings finds that we favor moderate complexity; a focal point in our surroundings; a moderate to high depth of field that can be perceived unambiguously; an even ground surface conducive to movement; a deflected vista, such as a curving valley; and little to no threat. While all these properties together "will elicit liking, preference will be even greater if a water feature is present."

Picture the Salmon River flowing across gently rolling countryside dotted with trees and occasional thickets of underbrush. Someone standing on either shore has an open view into woods or over clear ground. In either direction, the river runs straight until it bends out of view. This setting has a high preferability quotient: moderate visual complexity, a focal point (the river), moderate depth of field that can be perceived unambiguously, even ground conducive to movement, a deflected vista, no threat, and water.

We respond favorably to natural settings like this one in a manner that is bred in the bone, likely a heritage of our evolutionary past. The outdoor environment resonates with us, and we gain a sense of calm and well-being. As John Muir, titan of environmentalism and prime mover behind our national parks system, wrote, "Thousands of tired, nerve-shaken, over-civilized people are beginning to find out that going to the mountains is going home."

What Muir knew from experience, modern science has revealed through experimental analysis of human psychology. Two popular and related concepts frame the discussion of the benefits of being in nature: Stress Reduction Theory and Attention Restoration Theory.

Stress Reduction Theory

The theory that contact with nature reduces stress is grounded in the fact that our species evolved over 200,000 years in a close relationship with the natural world. As one researcher writes, "The environment that meets the biological and/or functional needs of human beings evokes preferences, positive responses, and a sense of well-being." Tests have shown that something as simple as a window looking out on a tree can have a calming effect on an office-bound worker, especially as opposed to one with a view of a parking lot. Even in small doses, nature is good for us.

Stress reduction from contact with nature appears to have far-reaching consequences for health. For example, a large-scale study in the Netherlands surveyed more than 250,000 people during visits with their general practitioners, asking them to describe their general health on a scale: very good, good, neither good nor poor, poor, very poor. Next, the proximity of respondents' homes to green space was determined using the National Land Cover Classification database, which maps land use in the whole of the Netherlands in 25 x 25-meter grids.

The results were clear. Those living in or near a green environment had better self-perceived health than people further removed from natural surroundings. As the study authors summarized in their findings, "Our analyses show that health differences in residents of urban and rural municipalities are to a large extent explained by the amount of green space."

Other large-scale studies have drawn similar conclusions. Researchers in England took health data collected annually from more than 10,000 individuals over 18 years. Subjects provided self-assessments of their mental health in terms of anxiety and depression, as well as of overall life satisfaction. Those data were then matched with percentages of green space where the individuals lived. The researchers write that their "analyses suggest that individuals are happier when living in urban areas with greater amounts of green space," even when controlling for income, marital status, and other factors that influence happiness. More green space meant lower mental distress and higher well-being, at small but significant amounts.

A Canadian study took an even finer-grained approach, comparing the health of Toronto residents with the number of trees on their streets, using questionnaires, high-resolution satellite imagery, and individual tree data. The results suggest that "People who live in neighborhoods with a higher density of trees on their streets report significantly higher health perception and significantly less cardio-metabolic conditions." These researchers conclude—in objectively rendered detail that is almost comical in its specificity—that adding 10 trees to a city block improves health perception in a way comparable to adding $10,000 to one's annual income or being seven years younger. More trees, more contentment.

Stress Reduction Theory seems persuasive on its face. Throughout history, people have found tranquility in parks and gardens, forests, and wilderness. Few should need convincing that sitting in your quiet backyard takes the edge off a stressful day. And whether our evolutionary past is responsible is less important than the reality we all can test against our own experiences.

A more complex, but at the same time more fascinating, theory of how spending time in nature improves well-being is reflected in a common and, especially in the present context, fitting command: Pay attention.

Attention Restoration Theory

We "pay" attention in the sense that we give it away, and what we give is a limited resource. It can run out. We are talking here of one kind of attention, which is called "directed" or "voluntary." We'll come to the other type, "involuntary attention," in a moment.

Reading these words requires directed attention. You must focus on the text and context, and you must inhibit distractions: external, such as the sound of a television; and internal, like thoughts about the weekend. These activities are fatiguing, as anyone who has studied for an exam can attest. Most of us cannot direct our attention for too long before we need a break.

To return briefly to evolutionary theory: Human beings evolved to pay attention to immediate threats and opportunities, not for prolonged concentration. We are, in a sense, as maladapted to paying attention for long periods as we are to living in high-rise apartments with noisy neighbors. Yet we do both, and each has its costs.

The fee for too much directed attention is fatigue, which leads to loss of focus and irritability. Modern human beings may be poorly adapted to directed attention, but we rely on it nonetheless and so must give it a rest now and then. A good way to do this is through *in*voluntary attention.

When we are presented with stimuli that are intriguing in themselves and do not require concentration—say, viewing a sunset—involuntary, effortless attention takes over, and directed attention has an opportunity to replenish. With directed attention restored, stress is reduced, and we feel relaxed.

Attention Restoration Theory, developed by Rachel and Stephen Kaplan in the 1980s, asserts that involuntary attention—what the Kaplans call "fascination"—is by itself not sufficient to rest our directed attention. Also important is "being away" from our familiar surroundings in a place that has "extent," that is, that constitutes an immersive experience, a whole other world that takes up all our (involuntary) attention. And there must be "compatibility" between the environment and our purposes; that is, the place matches what we want to do and offers all the information needed to do it. All these elements are found in nature.

Imagine going to a park for a walk. During your time there you are away from your usual unnatural surroundings in a complete world of its own, even, or perhaps especially, when the park is nested within a bustling city. The park is compatible in that it matches your purposes—you want to stroll, view the trees and foliage, and listen to birdsong—and requires almost no mental effort on your part. You are immersed in an experience that calls only on your involuntary attention. You are, to use the Kaplans' term, fascinated. The time away restores your directed attention, and you find yourself in a better mood.

Olmsted had all this in mind, without the scientific evidence, when he designed Central Park in New York. To shut out the sights and sounds of the city, he sunk below ground level three cross-town streets that run through the park and concealed them with foliage, and he placed trees along the park's periphery to obscure the view of buildings (he couldn't foresee skyscrapers). These features were meant to give city dwellers a respite within a green world at the center of a jangling, stress-inducing metropolis. There, the "occasional contemplation of natural scenes… in connection with relief from ordinary cares" was "favorable to the health and vigor" of New Yorkers, as it is today.

The benefits of attention restoration have been confirmed over decades by numerous empirical studies. A typical experiment has a large group of subjects perform a task that requires directed attention. The group is then split in two, with half spending time in a natural setting and the other in an urban environment, for a set time. Afterward, each group completes another demanding mental task, and the results are compared to judge the effects of each experience on restoration of directed attention.

For example, in one such experiment, subjects were tested with a backward digit span task, which required them to recall a series of numbers in reverse. The result was used as a baseline measure of their capacity for directed attention. Next, the subjects were given a 35-minute test to induce mental fatigue; then they were randomly assigned to either of two groups: One walked for about an hour through an arboretum, the other for the same time in a city. Immediately afterward, all subjects re-took the backward digit span test. The "nature group" significantly outperformed the "urban group" on the test of directed attention. And according to all subjects' responses to a standard test, the Positive and Negative Affect Schedule, the nature group felt better, too.

These results are typical and lead to a usual conclusion. Being in nature gives our tired directed attention a break so it can be restored. The experience leaves us in a better mood, refreshed and recharged, and ready to have another go at life's challenges.

Even more, restoring attention through contact with nature has proven therapeutic benefits. A famous illustration of this comes from a study by Roger S. Ulrich, published in *Science* in 1984, with the provocative title, "View Through a Window May Influence Recovery from Surgery." Ulrich was interested in varying recovery times for patients who underwent routine gall bladder surgery in a hospital in suburban Philadelphia. They were confined to hospital rooms for a week or two following their operations. Ulrich examined records for a sample of patients who underwent surgery between 1972 and 1981.

Nearly everything about these patients' hospital stays was the same except their recovery rates. Some took significantly longer than others to get better and go home, and Ulrich wondered if the reason was less medical than environmental, so he focused on patient rooms. These had identical dimensions and furnishings, all were on the second or third floor of the same wing of the hospital, and each had a large window.

The windows turned out to be the key. Some looked out on a stand of deciduous trees; others faced a brick wall. So Ulrich compared patients viewing trees with those staring at bricks, controlling for age, sex, weight, smoking status, and attending physicians and nurses, so that the patient experiences were as close to identical as possible. And he limited his observations from May through October, when the trees were in leaf. The results were remarkable and clear-cut. Patients with a "green" view were less depressed, took less pain medicine, and on average were discharged a day earlier than those looking out on a wall.

Spending so long in a hospital recovering from surgery is stressful and anxiety-inducing. Patients with few, if any, distractions are likely to brood and dwell on their conditions, just the sort of mental activity that drains directed attention and causes fatigue and depression. In the Ulrich study, those lucky enough to have a natural view during their recovery got a respite, a daily opportunity for involuntary attention to be engaged and give directed attention a chance to reset. Just seeing green had done the trick.

The green world celebrated for centuries in art, literature, and religion as a place of healing and renewal is precisely and provably just that. Fly fishing typically takes us to just such a world, like this trout stream:

The shallow creek runs swift and gin-clear over a bed of shale and limestone covered with a thin layer of sand and gravel. Stretches of the surface are as flat as a table, broken at irregular intervals by gurgling riffles and plunge pools. The watercourse travels through gently rolling countryside dotted by mature trees: green ash, black willow, eastern cottonwood, black walnut, and box elder, spaced far enough apart to allow a clear line of sight far into the woods from either shore. The ground is flat and largely clear save for occasional thickets of honeysuckle, buckthorn, and hawthorn. A fly fisher standing in the current looking downstream sees the creek far off arcing to the right and out of view, the vista closed off by trees along both shores.

The angler is well away from his usual surroundings—walls, hallways, clicking keys, beeping digital devices, chatting co-workers, the clock—immersed in a world of its own He is effortlessly attentive to the sounds of wind and water, to the push and chill of current against his legs, to the sight of mayflies emerging and a trout feeding and leaving its signature rise form on the creek's surface: a target-shaped rippling as though a pebble had been dropped into the water. For the fly fisher, the environment is eminently compatible. Nearly everything he sees matches his purpose and offers signs directing him what to do: Find a likely spot, select a fly, tie it on, present it to a rising fish. He does these things almost instinctually, thanks to practice and long experience; little mental effort is needed; he is fascinated.

The fly fisher's involuntary attention is fully engaged. No psychic energy is left to attend to other matters, to dwell on non-fishing problems. Directed attention is on holiday.

This time away immersed in a natural setting favorable to human well-being is sufficient to reduce stress, restore energy, and instill peace of mind. But fly fishing adds something more, a recuperative optimal experience—flow.

Notes

1. N. Frye (1991). Anatomy of criticism: Four essays
2. G.N. Bratman, J.P. Hamilton and G.C. Daily (2012). The impacts of nature experience on human cognitive function and mental health. Annals of the New York Academy of Sciences, 1249(1), 118136. doi:10.1111/j.1749-6632.2011.06400.x, 121.
3. Bratman et al., 121.
4. In K. Nillson et al., (eds), *Forests, Trees and Human Health*, chapter 5: Health Benefits of Nature Experience: Psychological, Social and Cultural Processes, 8.
5. R.S. Ulrich. Aesthetic and affective response to natural environment. Behavior and the natural environment New York, Plenum Press. I. Altman I, J.F. Wohlwill, 1983, 85125, 105.
6. J. Muir. *Our National Parks* (1901), chapter 1, page 1.
7. K.T. Han (2009). An exploration of relationships among the responses to natural scenes: scenic beauty, preference, and restoration. *Environ. Behav.* 42: 243270, 245.
8. J. Maas J, R.A. Verheij, P.P. Groenewegen, S. de Vries, P. Spreeuwenberg. Green space, urbanity, and health: how strong is the relation? *J Epidemiol Community Health* 2006, 60:587-592.
9. M.P. White, I. Alcock,, B.W. Wheeler and M.H. Depledge. (2013). Would You Be Happier Living in a Greener Urban Area? A Fixed-Effects Analysis of Panel Data. *Psychological Science*, 24(6), 920928. doi:10.1177/0956797612464659
10. O. Kardan, P. Gozdyra, B. Misic, F. Moola, L.J. Palmer, T. Paus and M.G. Berman (2015). Neighborhood greenspace and health in a large urban center. *Sci. Rep. Scientific Reports*, 5, 11610. doi:10.1038/srep11610
11. M.G. Berman, J. Jonides and S. Kaplan. 2008. The cognitive benefits of interacting with nature. *Psychol. Sci.* 19: 12071212.
12. R. Ulrich (1984). View through a window may influence recovery from surgery. *Science, 224*(4647), 420-421. doi:10.1126/science.6143402

Chapter 15

The Flow of Fly Fishing

The therapeutic benefits of optimal experience

"Flow" is the way people describe their state of mind when consciousness is harmoniously ordered, and they want to pursue whatever they are doing for its own sake.
—Mihaly Csikszentmihalyi, *Flow:*
The Psychology of Optimal Experience

The fly fisherman we met in the preceding chapter is standing in a creek born near the end of the last Ice Age, 11,000 years ago. The rolling landscape left by receding glaciers collected rainwater and snowmelt into small streams that swelled the torrent as it cut a groove in the earth. Fed by springs that keep the water cool in summer and relatively warm in winter, the creek remains open year-round. The water quality is high enough to provide drinking water to one community and sustain a large population of pollution-intolerant insects that live most of their lives in and on sediment atop the stream floor: mayflies, caddisflies, and stoneflies.

On either shore, honeysuckle, buckthorn, and hawthorn grow below green ash, black willow, eastern cottonwood, black walnut, and box elder. Nesting nearby are common nighthawks, red-headed woodpeckers, horned larks, golden-winged warblers, and vesper sparrows. The woods are home to whitetail deer, raccoons, eastern chipmunks, gray squirrels, red squirrels, masked shrews, beavers, woodchucks, minks, red foxes, opossums, and coyotes. On the ground and in the water are eastern garter snakes, red-backed salamanders, and snapping turtles.

Near the middle of this narrow stretch of the creek, a rock the size of an ottoman rests on the bottom. Behind it, a fish holds steady in the current, pointed upstream like a compass needle. It is a brown trout, *Salmo trutta*, its amber sides and dorsal fin flecked with dark spots and with dime-sized red dots running along the lateral lines. With a subtle fluttering of its fins, the trout rises several inches, opens its mouth, jerks its head to one side to gobble a bug as it rises toward the surface, and drifts back to its position downstream of the rock, watching.

For the trout, the creek is a smorgasbord on a conveyor belt. Some two million years of natural selection—*S. trutta* appeared in the early Pleistocene Epoch throughout much of Europe and was brought to North America in the late nineteenth century—have produced an exquisitely adapted opportunistic predator. Spending much of its life within a small range, the fish expends a minimum of energy to capture and eat prey that continually glide into view.

Now, in late April, all around the trout swarms of tiny insects are swimming from the bottom toward the light. These are immature mayflies, called nymphs. They attach themselves to the surface film, burst out of their skin, and emerge as duns, which resemble Lilliputian sailboats as they drift downstream for a minute or two to rest before flying off to trees or bushes along the shore. During their brief lives in the air, mayflies do not—in fact, cannot—eat: they have neither mouths nor digestive systems. They are driven by a single purpose. Within a couple of hours to a day, they molt again to become full adults, mate, deposit eggs in the creek, and fall dead or dying onto the water. These momentary beauties belong to the order *Ephemeroptera*, from ephemeral: literally, lasting no more than a day.

Mayflies arose some 300 million years ago; now 3,000 species are spread around the world. Their successful reproductive strategy is obvious: they emerge from a stream in a blizzard. All the while they are attacked, from above and below, by swallows and dragonflies skimming over the surface, by trout feeding on rising nymphs and floating duns. At dusk, the bats come on. But creatures swimming and flying cannot devour them all.

This display has repeated itself on the creek—previously with native trout that were later displaced by *S. trutta*—for millennia. Indigenous people watched from the banks, puzzling out strategies to take fish. They speared and clubbed them in the shallows and caught them in nets where the creek narrowed. They fashioned V-shaped weirs with rocks and branches to trap fish swimming downstream, perhaps driven by people spread shore to shore slapping the surface with hands and sticks. Perhaps mischievous children lay on shore with arms extended below an undercut, groping for trout to tickle.

The fly fisherman sees the trout's signature rise form as it sips a dun from the surface. Up and down the stream other fish are rising along a seam in the current, which draws the vulnerable mayflies into a feeding lane. The scene reminds him of Hemingway's story, "Big Two-Hearted River": "As far down the long stretch as he could see, the trout were rising, making circles all down the surface of the water, as though it were starting to rain."

Mayflies are blown across the stream and onto the man's face and clothes. He picks one from his shirt and inspects it. The size, rusty-brown body, and three tails, as well as the time of year, mark it as *Ephemerella subvaria*, commonly known as the Hendrickson. The dun's wings are greyish and dusky; after the final molt, they will look like cellophane. He selects an imitation fly from a wallet-sized box and ties it on with an Improved Clinch Knot.

His gear is the culmination of decades of technological refinements. His rod is made of microscopically thin carbon graphite fibers twisted and woven into a strong, supple material. His reel was machined from a single block of bar-stock aluminum and equipped with self-lubricating cork washers/discs to provide smooth resistance—drag—against a running fish. Between reel arbor and fly are fifty yards of Dacron backing; ninety feet of fly line, consisting of a braided multifilament nylon core inside a plastic coating; a nine-foot-long monofilament leader; and a short, wispy length of polytetrafluoroethylene tippet.

The angler wears four-layer nylon chest waders and rubber-soled boots with synthetic microfiber uppers tied with what the catalog calls "aircraft-grade stainless steel laces." His bulky fishing vest, its pockets crammed with fly boxes, is festooned with tools and accessories: nail clippers, hemostats, wallets for leaders and tippet, leather leader-straightener, fly desiccant, insect repellent. He has a collapsible wading staff on his belt and a mahogany-handled landing net attached to his vest and dangling between his shoulder blades. Clipped to the bill of his baseball cap are flip-down 2.5x magnifier glasses with a three-bulb LED. His outfit and equipment are worth well over a thousand dollars.

Planting himself down- and across-stream of the rising trout, the fly fisherman pulls line off his reel and lets it drift lazily away from him. He holds the rod with his right hand and the fly line between the thumb and index finger of his left, snaps the rod tip upward, and lets the line slide through his fingers as it reaches into the air behind him. When it is fully extended to the rear, he pinches the line and snaps his wrist forward, passing energy through the rod to its rapidly flexing tip, which shoots the line ahead at speeds of around 600 miles per hour. Line, leader, tippet, and fly roll through a tight loop until together they point out over the water, hang for a beat, and drop onto the surface. With an upstream flip of his rod, he mends the line.

The imitation now floating downstream at the end of the tippet is an Adams Parachute. Its body is thread wrapped with rabbit fur, its tail three microfibbets tied in at the hook bend. Behind the hook's eye, a stub of white calf's tail forms, perpendicular to the shaft, a post around about which is wound black-and-white grizzly hackle plucked from a rooster's cape. The fly, which resembles a helicopter more than a parachute, bobs on the water's surface like a newly hatched dun.

The trout peers upward in a 45-degree cone of vision, on the lookout for food and predators. Just as the mayflies are propelled to pass on their DNA, *S. trutta* is driven to eat, and now it is surrounded by food: nymphs rising and duns emerging and drifting above like an insect carpet. Hunger and caution push and pull the fish until it locks on an inviting silhouette and rockets to the surface.

———

Fly fishing is an immersion. Literally, as the fly fisher wades into the fish's element, but also figuratively. To be immersed is to be engaged, absorbed, engrossed—fascinated. Some of this engagement involves education and practice. The sport rewards immersion in stream mechanics, trout behavior, entomology, and the appropriate presentation of flies. Novices devote hours to perfecting their casts on lawns and ponds, storing line-management skills in muscle memory. And during time on the water, fly fishers are fully absorbed by the activity of locating trout and enticing them to take an imitation. All the knowledge and preparation pay off, if not in fish taken, then in the gratifying mastery of a complex skill. They stand in the flow of the current, immersed in the flow of technique.

In his groundbreaking book, *Flow: The psychology of optimal experience* (1990), psychologist Mihaly Csikszentmihalyi (ME-high Cheek-SENT-me-high) defines "flow" as "the way people describe their state of mind when consciousness is harmoniously ordered, and they want to pursue whatever they are doing for its own sake." People in flow are so absorbed by an activity that it "becomes spontaneous, almost automatic; they stop being aware of themselves as separate from the actions they are performing." In this state of optimal experience, a person is in control, free from worry, and elated. As Csikszentmihalyi describes it, the optimal experience has these common characteristics:

1. Intense and focused concentration on the present moment so that there is no attention left over to think about anything irrelevant, or to worry about problems.

2. A sense that one's skills are adequate to cope with the challenges at hand, in a goal-directed, rule-bound action system that provides clear clues—continuous feedback—as to how well one is performing.

3. A loss of reflective self-consciousness—no worries about oneself, and a feeling of serenity.

4. A distortion of temporal experience—so thoroughly focused on the present, hours seem to pass by in minutes.

5. Experience is so gratifying that people are willing to do it for its own sake, with little concern for what they will get out of it.

Csikszentmihalyi suggests that nearly any activity can become an optimal experience so long as it is something we are good at. Workaday tasks can produce flow if they elicit deep concentration that pushes all other thoughts aside as we become engrossed in what we are doing, confident that our skills are adequate to the job. Soon the border between self and activity dissolves; we are unaware of anything but what we are doing at that moment. We are so absorbed in the activity that we may be surprised to discover hours have passed without our having realized it.

Importantly, this experience does not require directed attention of the sort discussed in Chapter 14. When in a state of flow, we don't think about what we are doing because we don't have to think. We have the necessary skills and receive constant feedback from the activity to let us know whether we are doing it well. We proceed effortlessly from one action to another, like the ice skater in frock coat and top hat on the first-edition dust jacket of *Flow: The psychology of optimal experience.* As Csikszentmihalyi describes this experience, "People become so involved in what they are doing that the activity becomes spontaneous, almost automatic; they stop being aware of themselves as separate from the actions they are performing." They glide like an experienced skater on ice.

Flow is often associated with sports. We hear someone say of an elite athlete performing at the peak of his abilities that he is "in a zone," so focused on his performance that he appears unbeatable, like a tennis player winning point after spectacular point or a gymnast sticking every landing off a vault. Competitors in a zone appear unaware of everything but what they are doing with their bodies. A recent study of flow in sports and exercise describes the athlete's state of flow as "a full engagement in their athletic performance that involves an ideal balance among focus, enjoyment, the challenges of the competitive situation, and the athlete's skills."

The athlete's flow is a kind of peak *performance* in response to the demands of a competition with strict rules and expectations. In contrast with this is the peak or optimal *experience*, which unfolds more organically. A peak performance is focused and responsive to rules; a peak experience "is a transcendental, spontaneous, and joyful event that absorbs the individual into its moment."

Fly fishing is more experience than performance, with no competitive boundaries to guide or constrain the fly fisher's activity. There is no script, no step-by-step plan. Rather, the interplay of will and feedback—the fly fisher's desire to locate and catch trout, the information coming from the stream—determines the pattern of action. Csikszentmihalyi calls this interplay *emergent motivation*: "What happens at any moment is responsive to what happened immediately before within the interaction, rather than being dictated by a preexisting intentional structure located within either the person (e.g., a drive) or the environment (e.g., a tradition or script)." Fly fishers are implicated in the environment, in the movement of water, the life cycles of aquatic insects, and the habits of trout. Rather than follow anything like a script, they respond continually to what they see and hear taking place on and in the stream around them. The motivation to move the fly to another location, alter the drift of a line, or try a different imitation emerges spontaneously in reaction to changes taking place all around the angler: a floating mayfly dun sipped from below, the flash of a trout near the streambed taking nymphs, a rise form appearing repeatedly in the same spot. Fly fishers immerse themselves in the stream and in a peak experience.

Although flow can be achieved, according to Csikszentmihalyi, while engaged in many different activities, including working on an assembly line, truly optimal experiences involve doing what we love. Flow comes about when we use a skill with such effortless command that we enjoy a kind of ecstasy, an experience so intense that we are in a reality very different from the everyday. All that matters are the activity itself and the resulting sense of accomplishment and joy. Everything else, all the worries and preoccupations that fill our consciousness, melt away. The optimal experience is so gratifying as to be an end in itself.

The concept of flow developed decades ago by Csikszentmihalyi since has been refined and expanded in scores of studies, journal articles, and books. The experience has been broken down into various categories. In what follows, flow is applied to fly fishing using, with some modifications, the five common characteristics of flow introduced earlier: intense concentration, challenge-skills balance with unambiguous feedback, loss of reflective self consciousness, transformation of time, and *autotelic* experience—one so gratifying that people are willing to do it for its own sake, with little concern for what they will get out of it.

Intense Concentration

Fly fishers are singularly focused on locating and casting to trout and staying upright and balanced in moving water. Their attention is fixed on the present moment only. They concentrate on managing the fly line in the air and on the water as they present a fly to different spots, always on the lookout for signs of fish.

Intense concentration of this sort can and does lead to what flow researchers have named action-awareness merging, "creating a moment whereby the 'feeling' of doing is lost and the feeling of automatic response takes place." Like a trained and conditioned athlete, the adept fly fisher does not think about how to act but acts spontaneously. When a fish rises nearby, the fly fisher doesn't pause to consider next steps or to weigh options; she reflexively and immediately lifts her line and sends a cast in the direction of the fish. She is not, to paraphrase Csikszentmihalyi, aware of herself as separate from the cast she performs.

In this state of intense concentration, the fly fisher is attuned to her surroundings and reacts to stimuli without thinking. She is so engrossed in the experience, her focus so contracted to events within a narrow circle around her, that any irrelevant thoughts or worries recede from consciousness.

One fly-fishing instructor for Casting for Recovery describes this phenomenon as a moment when her "brain clears out."

"I'm not thinking about work. I'm not thinking about what stresses me. And I can see when the women are out on the river and fishing, they're not thinking, 'I'm a sick person' or 'I've got to go to treatment.' They're thinking about what they're doing and whether they're wading safely." As Sara (Chapter 6) said of her first experience of fly fishing: "I wasn't thinking about my next doctor's appointment or what was going to happen. I was just concentrating on the line and the fish. That's all I was focusing on."

Another breast cancer survivor and Casting for Recovery participant, Reina, had a similar experience: "On the river fly fishing, I'm trying to figure out how to cast and when that fish is going to come by, and I'm trying to figure out how to read the water. I don't have time to be thinking about anything else but that."

Sara and Reina were talking about their first time on a stream with a fly rod, when they had to do more thinking about fly fishing than the instructor, a long-time angler. Still, they found themselves immediately absorbed in the activity and remained in that state of intense concentration for several hours. Like other breast cancer survivors who have taken part in a Casting for Recovery retreat, they describe their time on the water as one free of anxiety and preoccupation with treatment. For some, this was the first time since their diagnosis that they felt this way. Their brains had cleared out.

Challenge-Skills Balance with Unambiguous Feedback

Flow comes when challenges and abilities are equalized. "In this state of balance, one feels both optimally challenged and confident that everything is under control." When a challenge is too great, the result is frustration and anxiety; too little, boredom and apathy. The sweet spot of the optimal experience is where someone is pushed to the limits of his skills but not beyond. He has a sense of complete control but is not preoccupied with how he is achieving that control. It is effortless and automatic.

With sufficient practice, fly fishers have the skills "adequate to cope with the challenges at hand," including matching the hatch to select an appropriate fly, tying knots to secure tippet and imitations, finding fish, making a clean presentation, hooking and playing a fish, and releasing it immediately afterward. The activity is goal directed, not only in catching fish but also handling the rod and fly line to make presentations, avoid snags, and maintain a natural drift.

Fly fishers receive continuous and unambiguous feedback from the environment while they are on the water. For example, they see immediately from the movement of a fly on the surface whether their drift is working. A dragging fly is easy to spot. What they see on and under the water produces a feedback loop that keeps fly fishers constantly adjusting their strategy, changing tactics until the environment sends other signals to change again. The fly fisher in flow is in harmony with the environment such that its clues provoke an automatic response.

With challenges and skills in balance, and with unambiguous feedback continuously prompting nearly unconscious alterations, the fly fisher enjoys a sense of control that builds confidence.

Loss of Reflective Self-Consciousness

We've seen how intense concentration on an activity when one is in a state of flow pushes aside all irrelevant thoughts. But worries and preoccupations aren't the only things cleared away. Completely immersed in and absorbed by the optimal experience, the person in flow does not reflect on himself as an actor, as the actions proceed spontaneously.

Csikszentmihalyi argues that our egos are constantly under threat and that we spend a good deal of psychic energy concerned about how we are perceived by others. "But in flow," he writes, "there is no room for self-scrutiny." This is because the actor's skills are matched to the requirements and challenges of the activity, and he performs automatically and well.

A fly fisher immersed in the sport's continuous feedback loop—moving from one place to another in response to fish or insect activity, adjusting his cast to accommodate the current, trying various fly patterns, always adapting—is responding spontaneously to his surroundings. The activity is so enjoyable that his ego is not threatened. Besides, fly fishers tend to be by themselves on the water as, according to stream decorum, they give other anglers a wide berth to cast and move about. Mostly unobserved, then, the fly fisher avoids others' critical observations and is left to enjoy himself without questioning how he appears to others. This loss of reflective self-consciousness leads to a feeling of tranquility.

Transformation of Time

Flow alters one's subjective experience of time. Typically, this is a sense that time has passed faster than normal. Completely engrossed in an optimal experience for a long period, we suddenly realize that hours have passed without our knowing it.

All veteran fly fishers know this experience. Especially when the fishing is good, they may continue wading in freezing water long enough for mild hypothermia to set in, so engrossed are they in the activity. But this is true for novices, as well. A Casting for Recovery participant, Leslie, recalls her first experience: "At first I was like—we're going to be out there for a whole hour? Three hours? What? I'm not going to be doing this for three hours. But once we got out there, time just flew by."

The flow of fly fishing comes about from the angler's enjoyable mastery and management of a host of consecutive activities while standing in moving water. That figurative and literal immersion so engages the fly fisher that he loses track of time.

Autotelic Experience

The peak experience is so gratifying that people are willing to do it for its own sake and regardless of any potential outcome. A special case has to be made for fly fishing, which does have an objective, that is, to catch fish. And fly fishers, despite their protestations that they are equally happy whether they hook fish or not, really do want to catch fish and are disappointed when they are "skunked." This is not to say that angling without landing fish somehow negates the experience. (As the saying goes, a bad day of fishing beats a good day at the office.) Much of the flow-inducing experience of fly fishing is in the metronomic sweep of the fly rod and mastery of line in the air and on the water. The total experience, even without a trout on the line, produces a gratifying sense of skillful command.

Fly fishers do often catch fish, of course. Otherwise, they likely would find a less expensive pastime. And the anticipation of having a trout on the line is itself a sort of buzz, a psychic ingredient in the totality of flow. The control of tackle, the attunement to the environment, and the expectation of success together constitute an optimal experience.

Of course, a truly optimal fly-fishing experience includes landing and releasing fish. With that final step, the fisher-stream feedback loop is closed, temporarily.

———

The rod bends, and the fly fisherman snaps it up hard to set the hook. In the trout's life, prey have never pulled back before. It flexes head to tail and back, forming a "C" and then its mirror image, so the line jerks and the rod shudders. The fish positions itself sideways to the current to be pushed downstream—and jumps, a blur and a flash of silver. The reel zings as the fish takes out line.

The fly fisherman backs toward shore and away from the swift current, pulling back on the rod and reeling in to draw the fish into the slack water. The trout tires quickly, and soon it is on the surface with one eye staring skyward. The fly fisherman wets a hand and cradles the fish, careful not to wipe away the protective mucus covering the trout's scales, lifts it just out of the water, and removes the hook from its jaw. Earlier he had crimped down the barb, so the hook comes away without resistance. With his left hand, he holds the fish nose forward in the current so water and oxygen wash over its gills.

The trout hangs limply for a moment. It sweeps its caudal fin languidly side to side, torquing its body so it nudges the man's hand. Then it slips unhurriedly away and stops where the man can watch it holding in the current.

Immersed in the activity that is its own end, the fly fisher checks his tippet and fly, drops them into the current, and when fly line and leader have drifted into tension, snaps the rod to the vertical.

If fly fishing has gained a reputation as a transcendent form of meditative engagement with the natural world, perhaps this is so at least in part because fly fishers appear to those watching them to be in a zone. And the anglers do often describe their experience as one of deep and blissful concentration. They enjoy a sense that their skills are adequate to the challenges of stream and fish, which offer continuous feedback on the fly fisher's actions in pursuit of trout. In this immersive experience, they focus solely on the fishing and become detached from not only any concerns or worries, but also their own egos. Enjoying the activity for its own sake and thoroughly absorbed by it, the fly fisher loses track of time. This is flow: consciousness harmoniously ordered such that the angler is serene, even elated. The optimal experience builds self-confidence and leaves the individual feeling renewed and refreshed.

Crucially, the fly fisherman we've been watching achieves a state of flow in a stress-reducing green world all its own and far removed from his usual surroundings. Completely absorbed by moving safely in the current, locating trout, and managing rod and line, the fly fisherman is in a state of deep concentration, so deep that his mind empties of anything irrelevant to the sport. Responding to cues in the environment, the fly fisherman acts more or less automatically, which gives his directed attention plenty of opportunities to rest. Later, when he leaves the creek to walk through the woods to his car, he is psychically restored and filled with a sense of well-being.

By providing an opportunity to achieve psychological flow in a calming natural environment, fly fishing is therapeutic for physically and emotionally damaged people. Of those, we sadly have too many.

Notes

1. L. Carter, B. River, B. and M. Sachs (2013, Fall). Flow in sport, exercise, and performance: A review with implications for future research. *Journal of Multidisciplinary Research*, 5(3), 1731, 18.
2. Carter, et. al., 23.
3. J. Nakamura and M. Csikszentmihalyi (2002). The concept of flow. *Handbook of Positive Psychology*, 89-105, 91.
4. Carter, et. al., 19.
5. S. Engeser, S and F. Rheinberg, (2008). Flow, performance and moderators of challenge-skill balance. *Motivation and Emotion*, 32(3), 158172. doi:10.1007/s11031-008-9102-4), 158.

Chapter 16

Conclusion

Take me to the river. Drop me in the water. —The Talking Heads

Cancer survivors, disabled veterans, and recovering addicts are alike in that they all have suffered physical and psychological insults. Many breast cancer patients and combat veterans have lost body parts; addicts, like cancer survivors, often have been deathly ill; members of all three groups suffer from post-traumatic stress; and every one of them is struggling to adapt to a new normal—sick, stressed, sober— that is surreal and disorienting. The future is not merely unknowable; it is menacing.

Reina, living with two cancers, worries, "There's always that thought in the back of your head: It can reoccur, it can reoccur."

Dale, struggling with combat-related PTSD, says, "A lot of times when I'm driving, I'll drift off and I'll think about what happened… It triggers anger and guilt."

Amy, while thrilled to be sober, still asks herself, "Why the hell, after being sober for 13 years, did I stop at a gas station and pick up a drink one day?"

Casting for Recovery organizers often say of the women who attend their retreats that it's as if they've been hit by a truck. That's a fair characterization of all the survivors in this book. They are rebounding from a hard blow. They may be optimistic about what lies ahead. Or they may see the future speeding toward them like a bullet.

As we've learned from many of the personal accounts included here, at some point all of these wounded individuals must move on with their lives, too often with little or no ongoing support.

Dr. Deb Norris reproaches those in the medical profession who leave breast cancer survivors to fend for themselves after surgery and chemotherapy. "OK," she says, pretending to shoo a patient out the door. "You've completed your treatment, you're cured, go on with your life."

Similarly, Bob and Merilee Hoover, while designing OASIS, were put off by the many one-time offerings for returning veterans, which may ease their transition to civilian life but too often leave troubled men and women to fend for themselves afterward: "Looking at other programs for vets at the time, they're all these one-shot deals, and then, so long until next year."

Jed, who is passionate about helping recovering addicts, knows the limits of that help. "They are on their own journey, their own path," he says. "I can't fix them or cure them. It's up to them. Nothing's changed out there. The only thing that's changed is them."

These three populations also share the indignity of being singled out as "damaged." The healthy look away, either out of discomfort at the evidence of their own mortality or loathing at the sight of another's supposed weakness. Whatever the reasons for that averted gaze, the result can be humiliation, isolation, and shame. This may be a greater unfairness than the damage itself. Reina brazenly confronted this subtle shaming by dispensing with scarves and wigs when out in public, practically daring people *not* to look, insisting on their attention.

Yet the voices recorded here speak loudest of resilience, despite the long odds some of them face. No one's outlook is more challenging than Sue's, whose breast cancer was metastatic when it was discovered. Nevertheless, she says, "I want to enjoy what I've got. I try to find ways to be happy." Sue could be speaking for everyone, each recalibrating his or her life to membership in a club no one wants to join: cancer survivors, PTSD sufferers, recovering addicts. They all are looking for ways to be happy, to regain a sense of well-being, to reclaim independence and control over their lives. They seek a new beginning—even those close to the end.

Each of the people we've met in these pages has discovered some measure of renewal through fly fishing. For some, that rejuvenation is tentative and fragile; for others, it is a virtual rebirth. Think of Reina recalling her ecstasy on the river when she imagined the water washing away the effects and memories of chemotherapy: "I hadn't felt so good and so relaxed in a long time… And I felt everything is going to be OK." The Casting for Recovery retreat was a turning point for her, as it has been for countless others still reeling from their diagnosis and treatment. She extended herself by trying something challenging and had fun for the first time since becoming ill.

When fly fishing is therapeutic, it draws the fly fisher into moving meditation during time away. She is immersed in the stream and the moment, watching for signs of trout, continually responding to feedback from the environment, casting and mending her line, absorbed in her mastery of complex skills in balance with challenges. That mastery is especially gratifying for those whose lives seem wildly out of their control. On the water, away from the ragged uncertainty of what each day could bring, they enjoy control and a measure of predictability. In a state of flow, they are elated.

And all this happens within a Green World. The space a trout stream glides through—with trees and undergrowth spread over even ground, moderate visual complexity, ease of movement—is itself conducive to feelings of well-being. Even more soothing are the sights and sounds of moving water. The Green World of fly fishing can be, as Rabbi Eisenkramer writes, "a life-giving place, one that… replenishes and nourishes the soul of the angler."

Fly fishing is a kind of baptism for Eisenkramer, as it was for

Reina when she had her first experience of the sport soon after completing chemo. She emerged from the water that day feeling purified and reborn.

The many volunteers of Casting for Recovery, Project Healing Waters Fly Fishing, and OASIS, and the counselors at Rainbow's End Recovery Center do not view fly fishing as a breakthrough or miraculous therapy in the treatment of shattered minds and bodies. They do, however, see it as an opportunity for those who are discouraged and depressed to discover they can still enjoy themselves. They are drawn out of their isolation into a circle of renewal, hope, and support.

In his groundbreaking book on PTSD, *Achilles in Vietnam: Combat trauma and the undoing of character*, Jonathan Shay introduces the concept of "moral injury," the profound psychological wounds suffered by soldiers in war throughout history who either witness or commit acts, such as the killing of civilians, that transgress their deeply held beliefs of what is right and wrong. A soldier could find himself in a situation—through what Shay calls "moral bad luck"—where he must make a snap decision under extreme duress, perhaps an immoral decision, in order to survive. He may feel betrayed by superiors who placed him in that situation and experience deep and lasting shame at what he has been a party to. Moral injury can splinter a combat veteran's worldview and destroy his character.

Treatment of this severe PTSD must, according to Shay, involve "communalization" of pain and grief. PTSD sufferers must be brought back into the community, where they can tell their stories to willing listeners and, through their narratives, "rebuild the ruins of character."[1] Crucially, Shay argues, we have a moral duty to support and face veterans with PTSD because they have served on our behalf. Further, we have an obligation to bring these men and women back into the community.

Therapeutic fly-fishing programs have this in common: They draw hurting people into a supportive and accepting fellowship that spends a good deal of time outdoors in tranquil, lovely settings. Besides being rejuvenated, these sufferers are brought into a new community. Casting for Recovery participants join a sisterhood of breast cancer survivors; disabled warriors regain the camaraderie essential to their identities; recovering addicts rediscover the world. All are given an opportunity to communalize their trauma and reset their lives.

This is what takes place when the men and women at Fort Drum gather at Remington Pond to practice their casts. With fly lines looping overhead above the lawn, the chatter moves seamlessly from casting technique to combat in Afghanistan, Iraq, and Vietnam to fly selection and presentation. A single conversation might include directions for completing a double-haul cast, an account of how an IED brought terror and chaos to a routine day, and a hilarious recounting of the time a few buddies figured out how to keep a vet's prosthesis from floating out from under him as he fished.

This communalization of grief and trauma happens when recovering addicts join a counselor at streamside to practice breathing in time with their cast. It happens when they discover metaphors in fly fishing that help them share their stories of loss and renewal with their own community of addicts and with those in the community they must rejoin.

When women at a Casting for Recovery retreat stand in a stream mockup to announce to the group where they are, metaphorically, in their emotional recovery—fighting for balance in the rapids, feeling less anxious in the run—they are building a new community. For many, it is their first time talking to others, besides family and doctors, about their breast cancer. As Laura Olufsen notes, "They very quickly recognize the fact that they all have something in common, and they open up."

Finally, everyone has the opportunity to join the community of fly fishers, as many of the people in this book have. It is a notably (some would say notoriously) exclusive club, a kind of secret society with its own idioms and etiquette. Those who join don't go through an initiation; however, before you can be accepted as a member, there is a lot to learn about knots, stream entomology, casting, and tying flies. Mastering these and other skills provides a sense of accomplishment that is a balm to damaged souls.

For some, becoming part of a fly-fishing group, either something formal like a local chapter of Trout Unlimited or a network of angling enthusiasts, can be an actual lifesaver. One disabled veteran who joined the OASIS Fly Rod Warriors told Dave Agness, "I fight every day to figure out a reason not to kill myself. This program saved my life."

Fly fishing always has been simultaneously communal and solitary. Fly fishers meet and talk and go to a stream in groups. But once on the water, they spread apart to a point where each is alone. It is a social enterprise, yet demands and cherishes solitude.

Likewise, therapeutic fly fishing mends singly and collectively. It helps suffering individuals restore fragmented psyches and broken bodies and gathers them into a community where the whole and the unwell make common cause in search of trout and well-being.

Notes

1. Shay, J. (1994). *Achilles in Vietnam: Combat trauma and the undoing of character*. New York: Scribner, p 188

Acknowledgments

I am thankful to many people for their assistance in completing this book.

From Casting for Recovery, I am especially grateful to Steve and Laura Olufsen, who invited me on the retreat that was the genesis of this project. Also thanks to Lisa Green, Dr. Joanne Hessney, Lise Lozelle, Dr. Deb Norris, Brian Ruscio, and Marina Swartz.

From Project Healing Waters Fly Fishing, thanks to Kiki Galvin, Daniel Morgan, and Michael Rist.

The organizers and volunteers of OASIS Adaptive Sports were generous with their time and information. Thank you to Lindsay and Dave Agness, Bob and Merilee Hoover, and Tom Tartaglia.

From Four Circles Recovery Center, thanks to Steve Hanna and Evan Snyder.

I am grateful to Nancy Del Colletti and her staff at Rainbow's End Recovery Center, who allowed me to spend a few days at their facility in Idaho interviewing counselors and residents and fishing in their pond.

Thanks to the anonymous reviewers of the manuscript and to Bruce Austin, director of the RIT Press, for his helpful comments on the text.

Finally, I am forever indebted to the numerous men and women—breast cancer survivors, veterans, and recovering addicts—who were so generous with their time and inspiring stories.

About the Author

Pat Scanlon is a professor emeritus in the School of Communication at Rochester Institute of Technology, where he taught for thirty-three years. He has published on a variety of topics, from Elizabethan literature to plagiarism to fiber optics. His recent articles on local history and fly fishing have appeared in several magazines. An avid fly fisherman, he volunteers as a river helper for Casting for Recovery, which offers free retreats for women with breast cancer. He lives in Rush, New York, with his wife, Joanne.

Colophon

Designer

Eric C. Wilder

Printer

More Vang
Alexandria, Virginia

Paper

Endurance Silk

Typefaces

Orpheus Pro
Brandon Grotesque
Adobe Garamond Pro

This book was made possible,
in part, through the generosity
of More Vang.